When Healthcare Hurts:

An Evidence-Based Guide for Best Practices
in Global Health Initiatives

Second Edition

Greg Seager

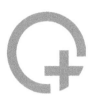

CHSC Publishing
201 Private Rd 5819
Grand Saline TX 75140
903-962-4000

Published by Christian Health Service Corps 08/04/2022

ISBN:
ISBN:
ISBN:

Library of Congress Control Number: 2012906534

This book is dedicated to the healthcare professionals who have chosen to spend their lives serving the poor through the Christian Health Service Corps.

All proceeds from this book are used to support the work of Christian Health Service Corps around the world.

Acknowledgements

T he evidence-based guidelines outlined in this book were submitted for peer review to the Institute for International Medicine and Health for All Nations.

Special thanks and acknowledgement is given to the following individuals who originally peer reviewed this material prior to publication.

Nicholas Comninellis MD, MPH, DIMPH

Jody Collinge MD, MPHTM

Arnold Gorske MD

Ted Lankester MD

Daniel O'Neill MD

Michael Soderling MD MBA

This book is dedicated to my amazing wife Candi Seager RN, who supports and shares my passion for brining compassionate healthcare to the world's poor.

Table of Contents

Foreword

By Ted Lankester MD

One person in five worldwide has no access to appropriate health care—that's almost 1.5 billion people. But in the global north our aid agencies and medical schools are generating an army of young people, ready to change the world. What an ideal scenario: vital needs being met by countless health care professionals, eager to move into action. Bring them together and global health is bound to improve. But is it? Most certainly not, says Greg Seager if we continue down many of the dysfunctional paths we are following at present. Right now many short term and some long term medical teams may be doing more harm than good. But, he goes on to say, if we get the interface right between the global north and resource-poor areas worldwide, the situation can be changed and the day can be saved. In this important and compelling book, the author from his wealth of practical and academic experience, talks us through the best practices which health professionals can follow to transform a global health movement from impending crisis to confirmed benefit. But for many who read this book it will be a surprising and difficult journey to make the essential changes he outlines. All of us involved in global health have to grasp the issues discussed here. If we don't, those with expertise, wealth and compassion will flood the world with good intentions. But in their eagerness they may destabilize health systems, undermine local health providers and cause increasing resentment. Against this backdrop Greg Seager outlines how if we get it right; short-term visits can be a benefit for all parties. Those working in resource-poor areas gain in their understanding of the world, and xvi Foreword poorer communities grow in self-confidence and competencies through appropriate training and encouragement. What needs to happen now is that these lessons and principles become mainstreamed into the approach and training provided by all organisations which send medical teams abroad. Greg Seager's book provides all the information and practical advice needed for these changes to be made. His approach meets the needs of the two essential reader-groups who have the power to make things different. Academics will find a meticulously referenced resource to improve practice and preparation in medical and nursing schools. Sending organizations will find a book rich in practical experience and stories from the field confirming the need for change. I read this book with relief and admiration. My hope and prayer is that it will make a vital contribution to all those responsible for preparing short-term medical teams so we can radically improve practice to the benefit of all.

Ted Lankester MD

Director of Health Services and
Co-Founder of InterHealth Worldwide

Preface

It has been a decade since the first edition of this book was published. Since then, thousands of individuals, groups, and organizations have used it to improve the quality of healthcare initiatives that serve the poor around the world. It is also being used as a textbook for global health service-learning programs in public health, nursing, and medical schools.

What has not changed about this edition?

There are two questions that comprise the underlying theme of the first edition of *When Healthcare Hurts* and continue to be a primary theme in this edition as well. Firstly, how do we create projects that support patient safety in healthcare delivery? Secondly, how do we respond to human need in a way that supports human dignity? The content of this book was geared around answering these important questions, which is the key to identifying best practices in global health initiatives. As we answer these questions, I believe you will find an interdependent relationship between community development work and effective global health initiatives. To think we can achieve best practices in global health work without a fundamental understanding of community development is a fallacy. Understanding community development is the foundation to building global health initiatives that build community capacity for healthcare, rather than diminish it —so naturally much of this book retains some focus on the community development practices.

As a side note, I use this word "development" because it is commonly used in cross-cultural work that facilitates positive change. I take my use of this word from the United Nations sustainable development and millennium development goals where it applies to systems and infrastructures—not people. The development I speak of here is about walking alongside people as they identify and overcome challenges to improve the quality of their lives. I do not mean it to imply that people need development. Without a mature understanding of these concepts, the meaning of the word "development" can morph into something paternalistic. We will look later in this book at breaking out of any paternalistic patterns of thinking that inhibit healthy cross-cultural engagement. For now, it suffices to say what development does not mean. It does not mean one group of people needs to be developed, and one group of people are the heroes that come to do the developing. When I use the word development, I am referring to a mutually transformative process where people from different cultures learn from each other, grow from engaging with each other, and together accomplish far more than either could accomplish individually.

What is different about this edition?

There are several things that needed to be updated in this new edition. For instance, since the first edition, the millennium development goals have transitioned to the sustainable development goals, and several of the educational resources and organizations listed in the first edition no longer exist or have transitioned their names and brands. This made it necessary to update resources and links to be more relevant. The most common critique of the first edition of this book was there were a lot of questions asked but not a lot of answers given. Because of this, I have updated the 6 Best Practice Guidelines listed in the first edition to provide more definitive direction and guidance. Although they remain conceptually the same, they are now stated with more clarity.

I have also tried to remove most references to "short-term." In some ways, this book represents the long-term perspective on short-term initiatives. Long-term workers are often quick to point out the flaws in short-term global health initiatives without acknowledging their own shortcomings. Long-term workers and their programs should exemplify best practices in global health as well. However, if we are honest, most long-term work falls drastically short of what would be considered best practices. Those working in global health long-term should put more forethought into patient safety, impact on human dignity, fostering a culture of patient safety, and improving healthcare quality—significantly more than short-term volunteers. This makes the precepts outlined in this book even more relevant to longer-term global health workers. There is a definitive need for monitoring, evaluating, and improving our global health and medical initiatives regardless of their duration. As such, I have moved away from a focus on short-term volunteers to include all those who serve cross-culturally in global health. You may still see "short-term" referred to, but far less frequently than the last edition. It has always been true the best practice principles outlined in this book apply regardless of a worker's term of service. They also apply to both secular and faith-based programs.

Much has changed since the first edition of this book, both in the world, and in my understanding of the concepts I outlined a decade ago. This is in part because I have continued as a student of global health initiatives for the last decade. I am a healthcare professional myself, and I am the founder and CEO of the Christian Health Service Corps. Christian Health Service Corps sends healthcare professionals from North America to serve the poor and build capacity of hospitals of low- and middle-income countries. This role has expanded my opportunities for study and observation of international healthcare programs. In the past ten years, I have visited many resource-poor hospitals and clinics in many different cultures. This has matured my understanding of these concepts I outlined a decade ago.

As of this writing in 2021, we are just emerging from the COVID-19 global pandemic, which has pressed the pause button on global health volunteerism. I am not sure if medical volunteerism will return to pre-COVID-19 levels, but if it does, it will probably take years. I hope that the global health volunteerism work that happens in the future will do so with greater quality and impact. Long-term work was impacted with patient loads and challenges of caring for COVID in resource poor contexts. However, most long-term cross-cultural healthcare workers stayed in place to provide care.

Medical and global health volunteerism seems to have shifted to a younger demographic with a bit more intuitive understanding of the need for global health engagement that is more supportive of human dignity. The book, *When Helping Hurts,* by Brian Fikkert and Steve Corbett, did much to reshape thinking around short-term volunteerism from churches in the global north. It helped people grow in their understanding of how charity work can build dependence and diminish dignity of the poor. This book, *When Healthcare Hurts,* addresses many of these same issues, but as they specifically apply to global health and healthcare delivery in low- and middle-income countries around the world.

Introduction

We were wonderful... or were we?

We made it! Our very first medical mission trip to Honduras, Central America. Days spent triaging, examining, treating, dispensing, and filling hundreds of prescriptions. **WE WERE WONDERFUL...**

Then, as we looked down at the faces of all the smiling children, we realized that the next outbreak of flu or diarrhea could claim many of their lives. We thought we were doing incredible things, but were we? We had gathered several physicians and nurses who would periodically travel from our church to serve the poor in Central America. This was a noble and compassionate effort, but in retrospect, there was much we were missing. Were our efforts of any value in the grand picture? Was a week's worth of curative healthcare really helpful? Our deep desire to help and to serve was real, but the one-week projects were really not the answer to the community's healthcare needs. As my wife and I began asking some hard questions about such projects, our eyes began to open to the grim realities of these kinds of global health initiatives.

The first extremely transformative event involved a Peace Corps couple who volunteered to assist us with a healthcare team in a rural mountain village in Honduras. About a week after returning home, I received an email from the couple detailing their deep regret for having been part of our "medical brigade." They outlined discussions they had had with the local population about how it makes them feel to see "the band of gringo doctors and nurses in matching t-shirts come to save the day."

Additionally, local health officials felt that the foreign medical teams traveling to the area were circumventing their leadership and authority. Perhaps most importantly, they shared their concerns about the safety of the care provided by volunteer groups, noting that these medical teams seemed to lack proper healthcare standards. The couple described how the patient safety and healthcare standards were much lower than those provided by local professionals. The people of the local community avoided the local health system when foreign health-care volunteers were in the area, thinking the care was superior, but in reality, it was far inferior to what was being provided locally.

Our group of volunteers was invited by a friend, who was a local pastor, and we had assumed there was no healthcare in the area. Why else would he invite us there? We realized we were deficient in so many ways, and the more we learned, the more deficient we realized we were. This journey of studying global health initiatives began by honestly asking one question: Are such projects potentially harmful to the communities they are called to serve?

We began to study global health initiatives from a different perspective —from the side of the receiving communities. We felt it was essential to establish how we were viewed by local health providers, the community, and community development organizations. We began by talking to local providers at health outposts and hospitals. Next, we spoke with personnel from ministries of health, medical, and nursing colleges, Peace Corps workers, and workers from several community development organizations. They reported encountering many challenges with volunteer medical groups, most of which we had never considered.

We learned from the Honduran Medical College (CMH) that there are between 2,000 and 3,000 unemployed Honduran physicians looking for jobs in any given month. Many physicians graduate medical school in Honduras and other Latin American countries, but, with little hope of gainful employment, go on to drive taxis and work in other fields. This is only one example of a long list of issues we discovered. Despite this, the airports in both San Pedro-Sula and Tegucigalpa receive at least one short-term volunteer medical team every day and sometimes several per day.

Sadly, we learned that there was a significant potential for harm in global health projects, primarily because of a lack of knowledge.

The Five Reasons Global Health Work is Harmful without Adequate Knowledge

1) Without understanding how to maintain patient safety in global health projects, there is great potential for causing actual physical harm to patients.

2) Without wisdom to develop intentional and effective partnerships, global health projects often diminish confidence in the local healthcare system and its providers.

3) Without cultural knowledge, global health projects are often paternalistic, offering crisis relief where long-term community development projects are the appropriate intervention.

4) Without insight into the local context, global health projects often cause economic harm to providers and health systems.

5) Without appropriate perspective, global health projects can be more about the volunteers than the recipients of care.

It should be noted, however, that with adequate knowledge even short-term global health projects can greatly benefit the communities they serve. They can help communities find answers to their own health problems and help develop sustainable healthcare delivery. Working alongside local health systems to plan and implement projects based on international standards, these programs can facilitate lasting improvements in healthcare delivery and the well-being of people. However, before we can help others improve, we must first improve our own efforts. We must enter a process of continuous quality improvement, learning and applying evidence-based best practices to our work around the world. This process starts by asking the right questions.

Asking the Right Questions

Have you ever returned from a volunteer medical project and wondered, *"What could have been done better?"* No matter how professional a program is, there will always be opportunities to increase effectiveness. The questions and case presentations in this book are not meant to criticize past performance. They are, however, meant to inspire thought on how to facilitate health development and improve the quality of care provided by global health programs in low- and middle-income countries. One definition of health development is "the process of continuous, progressive improvement in disease prevention and healthcare delivery capacity." When I speak of the health development process, I am speaking of building community capacity for sustainable quality healthcare and disease prevention services. Basically, it is community development as it applies to health systems.

Our assessment and study of global health initiatives began with asking one question about harm related to such projects, but there were many other questions that needed to be answered. The questions below are those that continued to burden our hearts throughout our years of global health work in developing countries. Although these questions were originally directed toward short-term volunteers, they are easily applied to any cross-cultural health care initiative. These questions have helped us and many others in the global health community define best practices. We hope they affect your work as profoundly as they have affected ours.

- Whose needs are you trying to serve? Is it your medical volunteers or the community your volunteers are assisting?

- Are you fully aware of the government and non-government health services being provided in the area? What is their capacity? Are you collaborating with them?

- Are you aware of the credentialing process in the country you are serving? Does each physician and nurse in your group have governmental authorization to work in the receiving country?

- Are the skills, knowledge, and expertise of local providers being acknowledged and utilized?

- Do your volunteers know and adhere to World Health Organization (WHO) standards of practice for low- and middle- income countries (LMIC's)?

- Do your volunteers adhere to acceptable pharmaceutical standards for dispensing of medications in low- and middle- income countries?

- How is follow-up care being provided to those whom you treat?

- Are the, heights, and immunization data being recorded for all children ages 0–5, and how is that information being used to support local health systems or long-term health programming efforts?

- Are you using the data collected by your medical volunteers to implement public health programming, either directly or through a partnership with another non-governmental organization (NGO) or governmental health system?

- What types of health education are being provided by your volunteers, and is it connected with health educators or health workers in the community?

- Are pregnant mothers being assessed for high-risk pregnancy and plugged into prenatal care where available? Do you know where and how to access higher levels of care for women who have high-risk pregnancies?

- Have you assessed whether or not your methods of conducting a healthcare outreach may be paternalistic and contribute to dependency?

- How can global health work affect the need for government investment in the health infrastructure in certain areas?

- Does your global health work adversely affect local physicians and facilities economically?

- If you are providing surgical care, are you working with a local counterpart to help build his or her knowledge and expertise.

After working through these questions, we realized the need for some basic standards of practice for health care work that serves the poor. Standards that would apply to short-term volunteer projects, university service-learning projects, and anyone working cross culturally in healthcare. We also realized that the standards already exist but are not widely known and are rarely used. This book is a core curriculum of best practice guidelines in global health initiatives. It is not this author's idea of what best practices should be, but rather a compilation of existing standards and guidelines that should be applied to our health work. I do, however, fill in some important precepts and principles that I hope will clarify the rationale for certain guidelines and standards.

Foundational Principles of Best Practice Guidelines

There are four foundational principles of best practices for global health initiatives. They are as follows:

1) Patient Safety

2) Healthcare System Integration and Collaboration

3) Facilitation of Health Development (assisting health systems to improve methods of safe and functional healthcare delivery)

4) Community Empowerment (helping communities identify and find solutions to their own health problems)

The first three principles of best practices are very much intertwined and overlap on many levels. They serve and support each other, and it is difficult to discuss one aspect to the exclusion of the others. Collaboration with healthcare systems and providers makes patient safety more achievable and can enhance healthcare quality on both ends of the collaboration. This, in turn, can facilitate health development by increasing attention on patient safety in partnering medical facilities and programs around the world. Community engagement applies to programs working at the community level to facilitate the community's response to its own health problems. This is perhaps a simplified summary, but it may help as the starting point for studying best practices in global health.

For those of us who send healthcare professionals to serve in developing countries, patient safety is often our biggest challenge, especially true for short-term volunteers. In the coming chapters, you will find tools, strategies, vision, and direction for your global health work, that can lead to better patient safety. Establishing systems and structures to ensure patient safety in global health is not without challenges. Our ability to create patient safety strategies is directly proportional to our commitment to quality improvement. It is also proportional to creating patient safety centered cultures in our organizations. There are a number of common practices and commonly held assumptions that represent significant barriers to achieving higher levels of patient safety in global health. We will outline six general best practice guidelines that address these barriers. All six guidelines included in this book are directed toward creating a culture of continuous quality improvement that both promote patient safety and support human dignity.

This book holds one underlying assumption, which is that healthcare professionals seek to <u>first do no harm</u>. We do our best to enhance patient safety and avoid adverse events related to the care we provide. The Institute of Medicine (IOM) defines patient safety as "the prevention of harm to patients," and they direct special attention to creating a system of care delivery that "(a) prevents errors; (b) learns from the errors that do occur; and (c) is built on a culture of safety that involves healthcare professionals, organizations, and patients" (Mitchell, 2008). The learning objectives for this book are, to a large extent, based on this IOM definition of patient safety.

Learning Objectives

Objective 1 – Readers will be able to identify systems, structures, and processes in global health programs that increase the potential for medical errors and adverse events.

Objective 2 – Readers will be able to identify modifications needed to facilitate quality improvement and patient safety in their global health programs.

Objective 3 – Readers will be able to articulate methods for participatory design, monitoring, and evaluation for their projects and programs.

Objective 4 – Readers will be able to articulate strategies for establishing a culture of patient safety and continuous quality improvement within their global health programs.

Objective 5 – Readers will be able to articulate World Health Organization (WHO) and International Joint Commission evidence-based guidelines and standards as they relate to global health programs.

Objective 6 – Readers will be able to articulate strategies for patient safety-centered partnerships that promote human dignity and facilitate health development.

Who Should Use this Handbook?

a) The guidelines contained in this book were written for both humanitarian and faith-based healthcare delivery programs that engage in global health initiatives (short-term or long-term).

b) Licensed physicians, nurses, dentists, pharmacists, and healthcare professionals of all kinds that work in and/or lead global health initiatives in low- and middle-income countries.

c) All licensed allied healthcare professionals that participate in and/or lead global health initiatives in low- and middle-income countries.

d) University global health programs, medical team organizers, administrators, educators, organization boards, or anyone who is involved with sending providers from wealthy countries to serve in low- and middle-income countries (short-term or long-term).

If you fall into any of the above categories, this book is for you. The guiding principles outlined in this book are about helping anyone serving in global health discover what constitutes evidence-based best practices for global health initiatives. However, it's not just about discovery of best practices, it's about application of them. In the chapters to follow, you will also find some strategies to apply these practices in ways that make a real difference in the places you serve.

This book remains relevant even as understanding grows around the need to promote and sustain human dignity in every kind of charity work—including medical work. There remains a monumental gap between the understanding of these principles and the application of them. We continue to see many of the same challenges and mistakes that volunteers were making when this book was first written. Few providers who step into resource-poor communities to deliver healthcare understand how to do so in a way that supports human dignity. Even fewer have considered or created effective plans to sustain patient safety while providing healthcare in poor communities. Understanding is the starting point, but there needs to be application with understanding. I believe many of the problems with global health volunteerism are that most volunteers lack understanding of how to work cross-culturally. However, application of these concepts requires more than understanding; it requires some forethought and planning. This edition of *When Healthcare Hurts* does more than just outline these concepts and ask questions. This version provides more of a roadmap for the application of these concepts, as *well* as continuing to ask important questions.

Even if you read the first edition of this book, you will find new insights and perspectives in this edition. I certainly do not know everything about global health work. I find being a student of global health is a journey of continuous learning—a journey I invite you to take with me in the pages to follow.

Chapter 1
Assessing our Work in Global Health

S ome may find this chapter challenging, but it is an important starting point: self-assessment. Do we, who engage in global health work, see ourselves rightly? We must be willing to look honestly at our motives and the quality of services we provide. As human beings, we are all broken, wounded, and deficient. We have no hope of helping others until we first realize our own state. We can say the same about the projects and programs we create to serve the poor. Our projects and programs are often imperfect, and we must see them clearly before we can change them. Before we can spark transformation in others, we must first see our own need for change. All of us have blind spots and weaknesses. In global health volunteerism, our blind spots are most often deficiencies in knowledge. Although, some are deficiencies related to attitudes and assumptions.

The starting place for assessing our work is assessing our motives. Looking inside ourselves, we need to honestly examine our motives for engaging in global health work. This is true for both faith-based and secular volunteers. Some people are motivated by their faith, some by a desire for adventure or recognition. For most of us, our desire to serve the poor comes at least partially comes from seeking fulfillment, meaning and purpose in life. This is important to recognize because it means we are operating from the top of Maslow's Hierarchy of Needs. We are seeking to meet esteem and self-actualization needs, consciously or unconsciously. Whereas most of those we are caring for are seeking to meet physiological and safety needs. This represents a different sociocultural divide that exists whenever and wherever we step out to serve the poor. We will discuss how this affects our work in more detail in a later chapter, but for now it helps us be clear about one question we all need to answer. Whose needs are we trying to serve? This question explores our reasons for serving in cross-cultural health projects. This is an important first step. If our efforts in international health work are primarily about making ourselves feel good, we have a problem. If, however, our efforts are about the recipients of care and not all about us, then we must place quality and safety as the top priority. There can be great meaning and purpose derived from serving the poor in low and middle-income countries. However, that should not be our primary motivation, because it can blind us from the potential harm such work, done poorly, can cause.

Maria's Story

A general medical team was serving a village community in Central America. Maria, a 29-year-old mother of five, arrived at the clinic pharmacy to receive her medication after having her entire family seen by one of the physicians. Maria had three prescriptions for herself while each child received prescriptions for parasite medications and vitamins. In addition, three of the children were febrile, and two had been diagnosed with otitis media (ear infections) as well as one with strep pharyngitis (throat infection). Each of them also received prescriptions for antipyretics (Tylenol) and antibiotics.

Maria waited patiently with the handful of prescriptions in the pharmacy waiting area. The line was long with about 75 people waiting for prescriptions to be filled. There were also people waiting to be seen by the dental, medical, and health education volunteers. Maria finally got to the pharmacy counter, and her prescriptions were filled by a pre-med student under the supervision of a nurse and a paramedic. The paramedic provided instructions for each medication through a translator at the pharmacy counter in front of the people waiting, all while Maria was trying to keep her children from getting lost in the crowd . Dosages were explained to her, and instructions were written in her own language for each child. However, Maria could not read. She received multiple medications in Ziploc baggies, rather than child-resistant containers, and took them home to her one-room, dirt-floor dwelling, with no place to store them away from her children.

Less than a week after the team left the country, Maria's six-month-old infant was brought to the public hospital in that region with acute liver failure and died. Maria had mixed up the dosages of medication and had been overdosing her baby with Tylenol for the entire week.

The Quality Chasm

In 2001, the Institute of Medicine (IOM) published a paper focused on closing the divide between what we know to be good evidence-based healthcare and the healthcare that is actually delivered to patients. This report remains as relevant today as it was over two decades ago. Its entitled "Crossing the Quality Chasm: A New Health System for the 21st Century" and it recommends six strategic aims on which to focus healthcare quality improvement efforts. They are known as the "aims for improvement," and they are: safety, effectiveness, patient-centeredness, timeliness, efficiency, and equity. Note that the first and most important of all, is patient safety. The IOM defines patient safety as "the prevention of harm to patients," and they direct special attention to creating a system of care delivery that "(a) prevents errors; (b) learn from the errors that occur; and (c) are built on a culture of safety that involves healthcare professionals, organizations, and patients" (Mitchell, 2008). If we take these concepts seriously in our home countries, we must take them seriously and apply them when we practice as providers in low- and middle- income countries. Global health initiatives have great potential to alleviate much suffering, but as Maria's story illustrates, they also have great potential for harm. Both faith-based and humanitarian volunteer organizations often enter the realm of healthcare delivery without recognizing the responsibility inherent in healthcare. As volunteers, we often get so caught up in the good we are attempting to do that we lose sight of the potential for harm that is part of any healthcare delivery. Returning home, ecstatic with a glowing feeling derived from our time of volunteer service, we define the quality of service by the quality of our volunteer experience. We too often look at the number of patients treated, and the number of prescriptions filled. We rarely consider the potential for harm that comes from such efforts, if patient safety is not a top priority.

As healthcare professionals, we agree that there is an ethical and moral responsibility that comes with providing healthcare from which no provider or organization is exempt. This is the inherent responsibility to provide safe care to patients. The World Medical Assembly puts it this way: "Quality assurance should always be a part of healthcare, and physicians in particular, should accept responsibility for being guardians of the quality of medical services" (World Medical Assembly, 1981). The question is, how do we achieve this cross-culturally? Healthcare—whether provided in North America, in Europe, or in Africa—has the potential to harm the recipients of that care. As healthcare professionals who engage in cross-cultural healthcare activities, we need to accept the responsibility of healthcare delivery to "first do no harm." However, this goal is not easily reached even in highly developed countries.

Based on data from the pharmaceutical suppliers of short-term medical volunteers, we estimate that more than 200 volunteer medical teams leave the US alone each month to go somewhere in the developing world. According to their annual report data in 2019, the leading suppliers of pharmaceuticals to medical teams, Americares, Kingsway Charities, and MAP (Medical Assistance Programs) International, together sent more than $1.6 billion worth of pharmaceuticals to low and middle-income countries (Kingsway, 2010; MAP International, 2010). They supplied a significant portion of these pharmaceuticals to short-term volunteer medical teams.

Clearly, providing medications to populations in need, or during a disaster, can have a profoundly positive impact. However, Maria's story shows how the dispensing of hundreds of millions of dollars' worth of medications in developing countries, owHowever hwithout serious attention to patient safety, is a recipe for tragedy. The significant volume of such projects, combined with the potential for adverse outcomes, makes establishing guidelines for patient safety and quality improvement in global health initiatives an operational imperative.

Challenges of Short-Term Initiatives

Concerns about short-term global health initiatives and patient safety were first published in "Short-Term Medical Missions: Enhancing or Eroding Health?" (Montgomery, 1993). In this older article, the author concludes that when such projects are assessed from the community impact perspective, they have little, if any, positive impact but considerable potential for negative consequences. Over the last 25 years, there have been several documented cases of child deaths related to short-term global health initiatives. Dupuis (2004) described two children who died in Asia undergoing cleft surgery, in the presence of severe acute malnutrition. One of the primary drivers of poor patient outcomes from volunteer care is emphasizing the number of patients seen over the quality of care provided to each patient (Garbern, 2010).

In 1999, Operation Smile, a high-profile and well-funded charity focused on cleft surgeries, drew much public scrutiny because of charges of shoddy practices. Critics charged them with putting the number of surgeries above patient safety for publicity reasons, leading to the deaths of four children in 1998, in addition to twelve deaths in previous years. In China, local medical professionals reported that 29% (which represents 169) of the children who underwent surgery by Operation Smile volunteers had major complications requiring ongoing care and surgical revisions in Chinese hospitals. These were not a few isolated incidents. In Kenya, a child died during surgery because of running out of oxygen, and in Vietnam, a child died from an asthma attack during surgery, a condition that failed to be uncovered in the pre-op evaluation (Abelson & Rosenthol, 1999). However, it should be said Operation Smile learned from their experiences, and they now have a significant focus on patient safety.

Any time we evaluate success primarily based on the number of patients treated, there is the danger of sacrificing safety. This is a concern for both short-term and long-term global health work since both are under the same pressure to manage sometimes overwhelming patient volume, and report to donors. Our most significant metric of success must be quality of care we provide, not quantity of care we provide.

What are the chances of someone being harmed by a global health or healthcare project? There is no way to know exactly, partially because little has been done to study community impact. I have reviewed over 100 post-outreach surveys assessing the impact on volunteers, but only a few looked at community impact, and none looked deeply at the idea of patient outcomes and safety. Bajkiewicz (2009), in his article, "Evaluating Short-Term Missions: How Can We Improve?" also describes the vast number of survey studies done on short-term volunteers and the incredible paucity of community impact assessments. The lack of patient outcome monitoring has left us in the dark as to the number of adverse events that actually occur as a result of global health initiatives. Operation Smile's adverse events came to light only after Chinese medical professionals, and some of their own volunteers, filed a long and detailed complaint to their board of directors. Charity organizations, that have experienced bad patient outcomes, do not publicize such events because it is just not good public relations and funding would be affected. It is reported that Operation Smile lost a ten million dollar pending donation that was diverted to another organization over the press received, in the late 1990's (Abelson & Rosenthol, 1999). However, global health initiatives are not alone in their lack of tracking patient outcomes in developing countries.

The Dangers of Medical Errors and Adverse Drug Events

The scarcity of patient safety research in low- and middle-income countries has in the past forced us to draw from research in from high-income countries. This has historically been how the World Health Organization (WHO) gathered most of the evidence base for its patient safety programs (WHO World Allience for Patient Safety, 2008). There is however a growing body of patient safety research from low-and middle-income countries that has come about in the past decade. Both the studies, from wealthy countries, and low-income countries raise serious concerns about patient safety in global health.

One significant challenge to patient safety is adverse drug reactions. They are among the leading causes of death in many countries (World Health Organization, 2005). One study estimated adverse drug events alone are estimated to account for 140,000 deaths in the US annually (WHO World Alliance for Patient Safety, 2008). At the time the first edition of this book was published, studies showed the number of deaths from medical errors fluctuated between 44,000 and 98,000 per year in the USA (Institute of Medicine, 2000). However, more recent evaluation of the data suggests the number of medical errors responsible for the death of patients is likely around 250,000 per year, or about 9.5% of all deaths in the US annually. If that is accurate, it makes medical errors the third leading cause of death in the US (Makary & Daniel, 2016). Some have argued the extrapolation of data was flawed in this retrospective study by the team at Johns Hopkins, and has served only to create distrust in the medical establishment. Regardless if medical errors cause 100,000 deaths in the US or 250,000 deaths each year, all of the studies points to one important conclusion. Medical errors are difficult to prevent, even in wealthy countries with systems and structures designed to prevent them. How much more likely are they to occur in resource poor healthcare settings? Studies in low- and middle-income countries is limited but here is some of what we do know.

Approximately, two-thirds of all adverse events resulting from unsafe care, occur in low-and middle-income countries (LMICs) (Jha, et al., 2013). 134 million adverse events occur in hospitals in low- and middle-income countries annually; this results in 2.6 million deaths annually (The National Academies of Sciences, Engineering, and Medicine, 2018). The occurrence of adverse events due to unsafe care is believed to be one of the ten leading causes of death and disability in the world (Jha A. , 2018). It is believed four in ten patients are harmed in primary and outpatient health care due largely to misdiagnosis and prescribing errors (Slawomirski , Auraaen, & Klazinga , 2018). It is believed 80% of these errors are preventable.

One study of ambulatory care in the US, showed that 1.4% of all hospital admissions were for adverse drug events (Jha, Kuperman, Rittenberg, Teich, & Bates, 2001). Another study described how 25% of patients who received a prescription from a primary care provider experienced an adverse drug event. Yet another study revealed that 5% of elderly patients, who were seen in the ambulatory care setting, suffered an adverse drug event (Gurwitz et al., 2003).

Much of WHO's patient safety focus has been on in-patient care. Since the first edition of this book was published, the WHO recognized the dearth of information on patient safety in primary care. In response to this information gap, they developed the Safer Primary Care Expert Working Group. The Working Group has published a series of technical reports on improving patient safety in primary care. In 2016, the Working Group published a report entitled, *Medication Errors: Technical Series on Safer Primary Care.* This report cited a number of studies that confirmed the need for attention to patient safety in primary care, as well as in-patient (World Health Organization, 2016). They cited, 12% of primary care patients in a UK study were affected by prescribing or monitoring errors, increasing to 38% in-patient over 75 years. It then increased to 30% of patients taking five or more medications (Avery A, 2012).

One study in Sweden found 1% of prescriptions had dosing errors (Claesson CB, 1995). Another Saudi Arabian study noted that about one-fifth of primary care prescriptions contained errors (Khoja T, 2011). The study from Mexico that was cited was probably most concerning. The researchers in Mexico found that 58% of prescriptions contained errors, with dosing errors representing most of that, at (27.6%) (12) (Zavaleta-Bustos, 2008).

What these studies make abundantly clear is that medication errors are a global problem. These studies cited, demonstrate medical errors are prevalent, even when care is being provided under the best of circumstances. Primary care, provided by volunteers in village communities, is far from the best of circumstances.

Based on what we know about volunteer run primary care initiatives in village communities, there is a much higher risk for prescribing errors in that context. This is especially true when those interventions and treatments occur outside of functional healthcare systems. Gorske (2016) addresses this issue in his article, "Why Patients are at Much Greater Risk of Serious Harm from Drugs in the Short-term Missions (STM) Setting—33 Systems Problems." He outlines common reasons dispensing pharmaceuticals in communities as part of volunteer projects places patients at much greater risk of serious harm (See Table 1).

Table 1. Why patients are at a greater risk of harm from drugs in the short-term mission setting (Gorske, 2016).

1.	Lack of understanding of the critical importance of the STM setting itself on the increased risk of serious patient harm.
2.	Lack of knowledge of the patient (Every patient is a new patient).
3.	Lack of adequate medical record, medication list, allergy record, list of diagnoses, etc. to determine whether a drug may be contraindicated.
4.	Lack of adequate time for obtaining accurate and complete history.
5.	Lack of adequate time/facilities for obtaining accurate and complete physical exam.

6. Lack of availability of reliable laboratory testing.

7. Misdiagnosis and inappropriate treatment of psychosomatic symptoms.

8. Lack of adequate provider training and knowledge of WHO evidence-based international standards and practice guidelines for patients of developing countries.

9. Confusion due to language and cultural differences.

10. Increased mortality due to lack of emergency medical systems and intensive care units for timely and appropriate treatment of adverse effects.

11. Lack of patient awareness of medicine's adverse effects.

12. Lack of package inserts, patient medication guides, black box warnings or other informed consent information legally required in the US.

13. Lack of adequate time for counseling concerning adverse effects by either the physician or the pharmacist.

14. Increased risk of drug interactions and drug overdose.

15. Disrupts the patient/physician relationship and continuity of care for chronic conditions such as hypertension.

16. Significant increased risk of accidental poisoning by STM children.

17. Increased mortality due to lack of poison control centers, emergency medical systems and intensive care units for timely and appropriate treatment of accidental poisoning or overdose.

18. Failure to comply with International Standards and Guidelines that require "There should be no double standards in quality," regardless of culture or economic status.

19. Neither the prescribing provider nor the dispensing pharmacist will be available when there are adverse effects from the treatment.

20. Local in-country health care providers and pharmacy personnel usually have little knowledge of our drugs and their adverse effects, and/or lack the resources to treat our patient's drug related complications.

21. Medications used by STMs are often donated and lack compliance with WHO international standards and practice guidelines for donated medicines.

22. Increased patient harm due to STM use of drugs which the CDC, AAP, WHO and other evidence-based guidelines report are of no therapeutic value and increase morbidity and mortality, especially in children.

23. STM use of drugs leads our patients to over-value them, resulting in additional increased patient morbidity and mortality, especially for children, long after we are gone.

24. Lack of compliance with International Standards and Practice Guidelines for the 70% of our patient's problems requiring health education and other preventative care.

25. STM use of drugs impairs and often delays local community health worker's efforts to resolve true causes of illness, resulting in increased morbidity and mortality.

26. STM use of drugs impairs local health worker's efforts to promote self-reliance, independence and personal dignity.

27. Because our patients are poor and drugs are expensive, medicines are often sold on the "black market" in developing countries.

28. STM use of drugs supports and increases the effectiveness of pervasive worldwide drug advertising.

29. In spite of our best intentions, the previously listed problems inherent in the typical STM setting magnify our drug-based system's harmful effects.

30. For the above reasons, the typical STM primary care setting provides a very poor teaching example for medical students and local health care providers and results in perpetuation of irrational use of medicines and resulting poor quality care

31. STM use of drugs inappropriately utilizes the placebo (belief or self-healing) effect, resulting in drug dependency.

32. Drugs as used in the typical STM setting do not support Jesus' teaching and holistic (Mind, Body, Spirit) approach to healing, but rather support a belief in drugs and magic.

33. Drugs as used in the typical STM setting also impairs the efforts of the WHO and our Christian physician missionary mentors to promote an evidence-based holistic (mind, body, spirit or Christ-centered) approach to healing.

Barriers to Patient Safety in Global Healthcare Initiatives

In order to improve patient safety in global health initiatives, we must be able to identify barriers that impede patient safety. Not having a physical infrastructure, through which to provide care, is often the greatest barrier. Many global volunteer initiatives attempt to provide patient care and dispense medications in churches, schools, or community centers, disconnected from any existing health system.

Seager, Tazellar, and Seager (2010) describe how this often leads to situations not conducive to safety. They cite the following examples: (a) non-medical church volunteers are often involved in filling prescriptions, and then instructions are given through translators by a nurse or paramedic; (b) caregivers of children may be given several prescriptions (usually in Ziploc bags) and often receive dosing instructions in front of a crowd of people, which can lead to distraction, confusion, and a sense of being hurried; (c) those same caregivers then take the baggies of medications home to a one-room, dirt-floor house, with no safe place to store them away from children; (d) patients often hold cultural beliefs about medicines that further cloud their understanding (e.g., big pills are for big people and little pills are for children, red pills are for blood problems and blue are for stomach problems). Dohn and Dohn (2003), in studying the quality of global healthcare projects in the Dominican Republic, state that as many as 36% of patients seen by a recent healthcare team had shared their medicines with one or more people, some of whom were children. In some developing countries, sharing medications is an extremely common practice with a prevalence rate of 55-66% (Beyene, 2016).

Providing healthcare in facilities not normally associated with healthcare creates multiple problems. The structure, processes, and monitoring ability necessary to facilitate patient safety are lacking in these kinds of locations. The WHO has established standards for patient safety that are an important starting place.

The patient safety and quality improvement model of the WHO was proposed by Avedis Donabedian, who is widely considered the father of healthcare quality improvement (WHO World Alliance for Patient Safety, 2008). This model is called the Donabedian structure-process-outcome model and has been the primary framework for assessing the quality and safety of healthcare for decades. According to Donabedian, three components are necessary for healthcare to attain any level of safety: structure, process, and patient-centered outcome assessment.

Donabedian (1966) defines structure as, the attributes of the setting where care is provided, which includes physical resources such as, the physical and organizational properties of the settings where care is provided (physical plant, money, human resources, organizational structure, and peer review policy). Process describes the actions of providing and receiving care, and outcome denotes health effects on the populations and patients receiving care (See Figure 1).

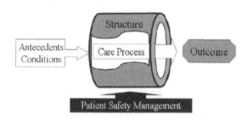

Figure 1. Patient safety management (Donabedian, 1980).

Can we achieve this model of safety in global health projects? The answer is yes, but not without some effort. Developing initiatives that incorporate this patient safety model inside functional, permanent healthcare facilities and clinics, is easier and should always be the first choice. Developing volunteer healthcare initiatives disconnected from existing health services presents enormous challenges to patient safety.

The impact of such projects on regional community development work is also a significant issue that we will discuss in later chapters. Patient-centered outcome monitoring, is a key to reaching an appropriate level of patient safety. Historically, this best practice has been deficient in volunteer global initiatives. According to the WHO Alliance for Patient Safety (2008), patient-centered outcome monitoring is considered an intrinsic component in advancing patient safety in healthcare delivery. Another important consideration is mutual design of global health initiatives, meaning local healthcare stakeholders need to be part of the planning and implementation of global health initiatives. This is foundational development practice which we will discuss later in this book in some detail. However, it also builds accountability and help often needed for patient outcome monitoring.

Mutual design, with local healthcare partners and medical programs, is fundamental to building capacity for patient-centered outcome assessment. However, disconnection from regional health system is not just a failing of short-term volunteer initiatives, it can also be said about charity hospitals and longer-term health programs. Long-term charity hospitals provide systems and structure to achieve a higher level of patient safety. However, if they choose not to have connection with regional health authorities and local providers it disrespects our health professional colleagues. Disrespect is not the a good way to enter and build a relationship. In the last 20 years, I have seen organizations from wealthy countries open hospitals in the low-income countries without including the regional health authorities or local physicians in planning. Four of these hospitals, one of which is in Central America, two in West Africa, and one in Asia, still have yet to hire their first local physician.

The cross-cultural nature of global health volunteer projects also presents significant challenges to patient safety. Providers may need to address regional, tribal, or sub-cultural worldview issues in their own homeland, as with an American physician practicing medicine on a Native American reservation. In many international settings, multiple cultural divides may need to be bridged. Providers may serve people from the majority culture of a country, or they may serve people from a minority community. It is important to learn as much as possible about the target community, not assuming that each country has only one language or cultural group (as this is virtually never the case). One example is where CHSC medical and nursing staff work in the Sierra Madre of northern Mexico at Hospital Mission Tarahumara. If a American physician wants to volunteer there and does not speak Spanish, there is a need for double translation. One to translate from English to Spanish and the other to translate from Spanish to Tarahumara. To provide care he or she must cross two cultural divides.

Another challenge can be care recipients' cultural beliefs and perceptions about healthcare and medications, which are often unknown to the provider. An example of a cultural issue typically not recognized by healthcare providers from wealthy countries is the selling of medication on the black market, that was received for free from volunteer medical providers. A mother faced with treating one sick child or feeding all of her children may sell medications to buy food. Clearly, language barriers also complicate understanding and can make instructing patients difficult. Dispensing medications is often possible only through interpreters, creating yet another obstacle to safety that needs adequate attention. Effective communication across the language divide can be a life and death issue.

Harmful Assumptions Impeding Patient Safety

Over the years we have discovered many widely held assumptions that impede patient safety and quality improvement. Being cognizant of them and evaluating if one holds such assumptions is essential to improving global health initiatives. Garbern (2010) described of the most prominent assumptions impeding patient safety, "Anything a medical team can offer in their limited time is beneficial." You may hear this assumption stated as "Something is better than nothing" (Dohn & Dohn, 2003). The second harmful assumption is that quantity is more important than quality (Garbern, 2010). Recall the Operation Smile problems of the late 1990's discussed earlier. It was alleged that the reported child deaths directly resulted from too much attention paid to quantity of cases and too little attention paid to healthcare quality. The one volunteer who wrote the board of directors reportedly asked an important question that all programs and volunteers need to ask: "Why do we not employ the same standards of care on missions as we do in our home countries?" (Abelson & Rosenthol, 1999). It is difficult to overcome this hurdle because global health charity programs (faith-based and humanitarian) draw funding from outside sources and counting numbers of patients and prescriptions is the typical fundraising model for many global healthcare initiatives. A quick search of healthcare mission opportunities on the web shows how we define success. One site after another reports the number of patients treated and the number of volunteers taking part, yet very few have any reference to patient safety or their healthcare quality assurance programs. Almost universally, international medical charity programs, from the largest to the smallest, define their success to the public by quantity, not quality. Not that counting numbers for reporting is unacceptable for public relations; it is a normal and acceptable practice in fundraising. However, the internal program question must be: Which has the higher priority, patient safety or the volume of patients treated and volunteers deployed? If patient safety is not the answer, then fundamental change needs to occur. What this change should look like and how it can be achieved will be discussed in the following chapters.

References

Abelson, R., & Rosenthol, E. (1999, November 24). *Charges of shoddy practice taint gifts of plastic surgery.* Retrieved December 1, 2011, from New York Times World: http://www.nytimes.com/1999/11/24/world/charges-of-shoddy-prac-tices-taint-gifts-of-plastic-surgery.html?pagewanted=print&src=pm

Avery A, B. N. (2012). *Investigating the Prevalence and Causes of Prescribing Errors in General Practice: The Practice Study.* London: General Medical Council.

Bajkiewicz, C. (2009). Evaluating short-term missions: how can we improve. *The Journal of Christian Nursing,* 110-114.

Claesson CB, B. K. (1995). Prescription Errors Detected by Swedish Pharmacists. *International Journal of Pharmacy Practice,* 3:151-6.

Dohn, M. N., & Dohn , A. L. (2003). Quality of care on short term medical missions: experience with a standardized medical record and related issues. *Missiology: An International Review* , 417-429.

Donabedian, A. (1966). Evaluating the Quality of Medical Care. *The Milbank Memorial Fund Quarterly, 44*(3), 166-203.

Donabedian, A. (1980). *Explorations in quality assessment and monitoring; the definition of quality and approaches to its assessment.* Ann Arbor, MI: Health Administration Press.

Dupuis, C. (2004). Humanitarian missions in the Third World. *Journal of Plastic and Reconstructive Surgery,* 433-35.

Garbern, S. C. (2010). Medical relief trips...whats missing? Exploring the ethical issues and the physician-patient relationship. *Einstein Journal of Biology and Medicine,* 38-40.

Gurwitz, J. H., Field, T. S., Harold, L. R., Rothschild, J., Debellis, K., Seger, A. C., . . . Bates, D. W. (2003). Incidence and preventability of adverse drug events among older person in the ambulatory care setting. *Journal of the American Medical Association*, 1107-1116.

Institute of Medicine . (2000). *To err is human.* Washington D.C. : National Academy Press .

Institute of Medicine. (2001). *Crossing the quality chasm.* Washington D.C.: National Academy Press.

Jha, A. K., Kuperman, G. J., Rittenberg, E., Teich, J. M., & Bates, D. W. (2001). Identifying hospital admissions due to adverse drug events using a computer based monitor. *Journal of Pharmacoepidemiology*, 113-119.

Khoja T, N. Y. (2011). Medication Errors in Primary Care in Riyadh City, Saudi Arabia. *Eastern Mediterranean Health Journal*, 17:156-9.

Kingsway Charities. (2010). *Kingswaycharities Annual Reports.* Retrieved December 7, 2011, from http://www.kingswaycharities.org/index.php/about/annual-reports/

MAP International . (2010). *MAP Financial Reports.* Retrieved December 7, 2010, from Map International : http://www.map.org/we-are-map/about-map/financial/

Mitchell, P. H. (2008, April). *Chapter 1 Patient Safety and Quality: An Evidence-Based Handbook for Nurses Patient Safety.* (R. G. Hughes, Ed.) Retrieved October 5th, 2011, from www.ahrq.gov: http://www.ahrq.gov/qual/nurseshdbk/

Montgomery, L. M. (1993). Short term missions: enhancing or eroding health? . *Missiology* , 333-331.

Seager, G. D., Tazellar, G., & Seager, C. D. (2010). The perils and promise of short term healthcare missions . *Journal of Christian Nursing* , 262-266.

WHO Alliance for Patient Safety. (2008). *Implementation manual for surgical safety checklist.* Geneva: WHO Alliance for Patient Safety.

WHO World Alliance for Patient Safety. (2008). *Summary of the evidence on patient safety.* 2008: WHO World Alliance for Patient Safety.

World Health Organization. (2005). *The safety of medicines; fact sheet 293.* Retrieved September 21, 2011, from WHO : http://www.who.int/mediacentre/factsheets/fs293/en/

World Health Organization. (2016). *Medication Errors: Technical Series on Safer Primary Care.* Geneva.

World Medical Assembly. (1981, October). *WMA Lisbon declaration on rights of patients.* Retrieved October 3, 2011, from World Medical Association: http://www.wma.net/en/30publications/10policies/l4/

Zavaleta-Bustos, M. L.-P.-H.-L.-C. (2008). Prescription Errors in a Primary Care University Unit: Urgency of Pharmeceutical Care in Mexico. *Revista Brasileira De Ciências Farmacêuticas,* 44:115-25.

Stuff to fix on this chapter:

• The IOM section

• The structure-process-outcome model section

• The reference to Dohn and Dohn 36%

• The bibliography to make sure it is current and accurate

Chapter 2
In Pursuit of Excellence

"Excellence is never an accident; it is the result of high intention, sincere effort, intelligent direction, skillful execution and the vision to see obstacles as opportunities."

- Anonymous

In Pursuit of Excellence

The global health guidelines presented in this book are based primarily on World Health Organization (WHO) directives, since they remain the global authority on health and international health policy. They were also developed based on guidelines from other agencies that have the authority to speak to patient safety and healthcare quality improvement including the United Nations International Children's Emergency Fund (UNICEF), Institute for Healthcare Improvement (IHI), and Joint Commission International. In 2005, WHO designated the Joint Commission International as the "WHO collaborating center for patient safety solutions" because they are a world-recognized leader in patient safety. IHI is also an internationally recognized organization working to improve healthcare quality and patient safety globally. The focus of most of the guidelines is patient safety. The challenge in the development of these guidelines was extrapolating applicable key concepts from the voluminous amount of WHO, UNICEF, IHI, and Joint Commission International evidence geared toward permanent health facilities and ambulatory care centers. The healthcare delivery guidelines listed in this book are exactly that: a compilation of key points from core patient safety documents of the WHO, UNICEF, Joint Commission International, and IHI as they apply to global health initiatives.

It is important to remember that all the agencies listed above have created standards and guidelines for permanent healthcare facilities. We must cautiously consider how and what standards can be applied to short-term healthcare projects and what impact the application of those standards will have on patient safety related to such projects. There are some rare circumstances in which the blanket application of documents meant for permanent health centers can impede patient safety in short-term global health projects. We will discuss this in greater detail in later chapters. *Accreditation Standards for Primary Care Centers* is a good example of this, probably representing the most applicable current published standards for primary care global health projects (Joint Commission International, 2008). They are excellent standards that affirm best evidence-based healthcare delivery, but they assume that patient safety programs are already an integral part of the primary healthcare center. This is often not the case in short-term global health programs, so caution must be exercised in application to short-term initiatives. Without significant experience in implementing global health projects, it is difficult to select which sections should be applied and which should not. They all apply in one way or another to permanent healthcare delivery programs in the low and middle-income countries. Whether they are achievable in poor communities is another question entirely. Our organization CHSC, comes alongside organizations with whom we partner to help them define their goals and what is achievable. In many instances it is not realistic to raise resource poor facilities and programs to the "gold standard" of healthcare delivery. However, some improvement is always possible, we can always work toward a "Silver standard". That is why we call our quality improvement support program "Iron to Silver". We seek to help health programs in resource poor communities at least aspire toward a silver standard, even if the gold standard is out of their reach. We also believe short-term volunteer driven healthcare initiatives can do the same, look to achieving at least a silver standard of healthcare quality.

Many of the standards outlined by WHO, and UNICEF do directly apply with little or no modification. The challenge is few healthcare professionals trained in wealthy countries know these standards exist let alone how to implement them. Here are a few examples of standards health professionals trained in wealthy countries need to learn before practicing in a low or middle-income country.

The WHO/UNICEF program, Integrated Management of Childhood Illness (IMCI), presents the internationally recognized standards for outpatient healthcare for children (0–5 years of age) in resource poor settings. Also, The *WHO Child Growth Standards and the Identification of Severe Acute Malnutrition in Infants and Children* is an essential document for all providers seeing pediatric patients in developing countries. It outlines the international assessment and classification standards for childhood malnutrition (WHO, 2009). These are primary standards that should be incorporated by all global healthcare programs. The WHO Surgical Safety Program sets forth the standards for surgical practice in developing countries (WHO World Alliance for Patient Safety, 2009).

Other attempts at guideline development include the Volunteers in Pediatric Plastic Surgery patient safety guidelines that have been reviewed and approved by the American Association of Plastic Surgeons, the Plastic Surgery Education Foundation, and the Society for Pediatric Anesthesia (Schneider et al.,2011). These standards are not based on WHO recommendations to improve patient safety. They do not recognize the WHO Surgical Safety Program, but they offer some key cross-cultural insights not addressed by WHO that need to be included for international programs. This will be discussed in more detail in a later Chapter.

Guidelines for developing training experiences in global health are another area of concern; however, these guidelines only address them in relation to patient safety. Crump, Sugarman, and the Working Group on Global Health Training (2010), in their article "Global health training: Ethics and best guidelines for training experiences in global health," outline some additional key guidelines for international global health training. There have also been guidelines created in the area of community-based global health initiatives for screenings and health education (Gorske, 2011).

It is ok to use articles written on this topic to get ideas on how to improve safety, but be cautious if they are not evidence based and only represent someone's opinion. The best practice guidelines outlined in the following chapters were developed to help guide policy development for programs providing healthcare in developing countries. They are not meant to dictate specific regulations for global health programs. There is a growing body of literature about best practices in global health initiatives. Some of it is good evidence based practice, some of it is opinion from people who have no full-time global health experience.

Lasker, et al., (2018) analyzed 27 guidelines extracted from a literature review performed in 2017. Attention was given to guidelines proposed and implemented by "short-term medical missions (STMMs)" and outline in the literature. They also considered how these guidelines correlated to the expectations of host communities, and host country staff who work with volunteers. Their results were no surprise. First, existing guidelines are almost entirely written by practitioners and educators in the global north with limited or no full-time global health experience. However, amongst the guidelines proposed in 27 articles there was consensus on key principles for responsible and ethical cross-cultural global health engagement. The need for host partners, proper preparation and supervision of volunteers, needs assessment and evaluation, sustainability, and adherence to pertinent legal and ethical standards.

Host country staff assessments do align with guideline consensus. However, they added the importance of mutual learning and respect for hosts. As a student of global health activities for decades now, this stands out to me the most. The consensus for standards in global health activities by volunteers from wealthy countries failed to prioritize the importance of mutual learning and respect. Nearly all the articles written to propose guidelines for short-term volunteers, are by short-term volunteer. Without a multi-cultural perspective involving local providers and long-term global health workers, the development of such guidelines is inherently flawed. Without looking to already established standards by organizations like WHO, and UNICEF such efforts will likely not be evidenced-based. And without a relief and development perspective they will fail to support human dignity in the context of responding to human need.

This book, and the previous version does not theorize new standards and guidelines for global health engagement. It highlights and discusses standards and guidelines that already exist from WHO, UNICEF, International Joint Commission, IHI, and the relief and development community.

The relief and development community has created a set of comprehensive minimum standards for humanitarian response, although they have been slow to make significant progress in the USA. These standards, known as the Sphere standards, are a set of principles and minimum standards created to improve quality and accountability of humanitarian response in four technical areas: Water supply, sanitation, and hygiene promotion (WASH), Food security and nutrition, Shelter and settlement, and last but not least Health.

Sphere was founded in 1997, as a collaborative effort amongst more than 300 relief and development agencies. This unprecedented effort came about after the humanitarian community recognized that better organization and collaboration could have saved thousands of lives during the Rwandan genocide of the 1990's. Today, the Sphere standards have become the foundation of disaster and refugee response globally. The Sphere Handbook is the primary reference tool in humanitarian crisis used by relief and development organizations, advocacy groups, governments, Red Cross Red Crescent, United Nations, World Food Program, etc. It puts all the organizations responding to an international crisis in the same playbook and holds them all accountable to the same agreed upon minimum standards.

There are multiple standards in each technical sector: Water supply, sanitation, and hygiene promotion (WASH), Food security and nutrition, Shelter and settlement, and Health. Each standard has a list of key actions, key indicators, and guidance notes recognizing it is not always possible to achieve the standards fully. All of the standards were created around the Humanitarian Charter and the Protection Principles. The Humanitarian Charter is part statement of established legal rights and obligations, and part a statement of shared beliefs of the relief and development community. The Charter is the legal and ethical framework for the Protection Principles, the Core Humanitarian Standard and the Minimum Standards that are outlined by Sphere. The Humanitarian

Charter is centered around three primary human rights and it applies broadly to all types of relief and development work including medical work. These rights are: the right to life with dignity, the right to receive humanitarian assistance, and the right to protection and security.

There are Four Protection Principles, and they apply to all humanitarian action by any and all humanitarian actors. The Protection Principles are: *1) Enhance the safety, dignity and rights of people, and avoid exposing them to harm. 2) Ensure people's access to assistance according to need and without discrimination. 3) Assist people to recover from the physical and psychological effects of threatened or actual violence, coercion or deliberate deprivation. 4) Help people claim their rights* (Sphere Association, 2018).

These rights and principles were created for relief and development organizations working primarily in crisis situations, but they also apply to any global health activities. Response to human need in any context requires guidance and intentionality to support human dignity, not diminish it.

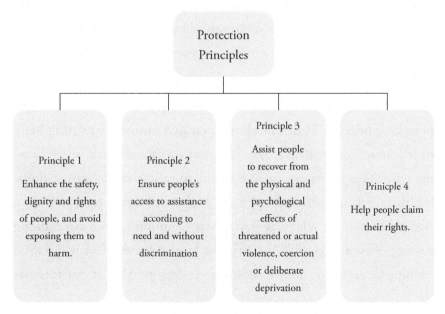

(Sphere Association, 2018)

Another core document upon which the sphere standards are built is the International Red Cross Red Crescent Code of Conduct (Sphere Association, 2018). This code was created to establish standards of conduct and behavior to which all organizations should adhere. It too was developed with input from a large portion of the relief and development community. Most non-governmental organizations (NGO's) responding to disasters have signed the Code of Conduct, it applies to both faith-based and secular organizations. There is much within the Sphere Minimum Standards, the Humanitarian Charter, the Protection Principles, and the International Code of Conduct that apply to global health work. They provide foundational understanding of how to respond to human need in a way the supports and promotes human dignity. Understanding the Humanitarian Charter, the Protection Principles, and the Health Sector minimum standards is a good starting place for entry into global health initiatives.

These principles apply to all global health initiatives and cross-cultural medical work because at the center of them is the consideration of human dignity. It forces us to ask questions about how our work respects the dignity of both our partners and recipients of our care.

In fact, Principle 1 (Enhance the safety, dignity and rights of people, and avoid exposing them to harm) is the foundation the best practice guidelines in this book were created out of the existing body of literature and evidence. Building on this foundation, the following guidelines are meant to address the most critical aspects of global health initiatives, i.e. those with the highest potential for harm. As a side note, there are relatively few Sphere Minimum Standards training courses offered in the USA. Christian Health Service Corps (CHSC) training department does at least one course per year at our international operations center in Grand Saline Texas. You can find out more on the training section of our website www.healthservicecorps.org.

As mentioned in the beginning of this chapter, we consider the final authority over international healthcare to reside with the World Health Organization (WHO). However, there are many issues in global health that are not directly addressed by WHO. Issues dealing with development aspects of global health projects not addressed by the WHO, such as respecting the dignity of our patients and local colleagues, we need to look to other sources. In those areas we look to the relief and development community and standards such as LEAP (Learning through Evaluation, Accountability & Planning) and Sphere which we discussed here. We will discuss LEAP in more detail in later chapters.

All six guidelines are presented here in summary, but we will discuss each in detail with the accompanying rationales in the chapters to follow.

Best Practice Guideline 1 – Build a Patient Safety Centered Organizational Culture

Best Practice Guideline 2 – Go as Learner, not as Teacher

Best Practice Guideline 3 – Practice Patient Safety

Best Practice Guideline 4 – Document All Care Provided

Best Practice Guideline 5 – Build Capacity for Health

Best Practice Guideline 6 – Design, Monitor, and Evaluate Projects Using Participatory Methods

References

Crump, J. A., & Sugarman, J. (2010). Global health training: Ethics and best guidelines for training experiences in global health. *Journal of the American Society of Tropical Medicine and Hygiene*, 1178-1182.

Gorske, A. (2011). Evidence based community health screening and education guidelines. *HEPFDC*. Retrieved from http://hepfdc.info/files/CHSEGuide.pdf

Joint Commission International. (2008). *Accreditation standards for primary care centers*. Oak Brook, IL: Joint Commission International.

Lasker, J. N., Aldrink , M., Balasubramaniam, R., Caldron, P., Compton, B., Evert, J., . . . Siegel, S. (2018). Guidelines for responsible short-term global health activities: developing common principles. *Globalization and Health*, 1-9. doi:DOI 10.1186/s12992-018-0330-4

Schneider, W. J., Politis, G. D., Gosain, A. K., Migliori, M. R., Cullington, J. R., & Peterson, E. L. (2011). Volunteers in plastic surgery guidelines for providing surgical care of children in the less developed world. *Journal of Plastic and Reconstructive Surgery*, 2477-2486.

Sphere Association. (2018). *The Sphere Handbook: Humanitarian Charter and Minimum Standards in Humanitarian Response, fourth edition*. Geneva, Switzerland: Sphere Association. Retrieved from https://www.spherestandards.org/handbook/

WHO World Alliance for Patient Safety. (2009). *WHO Guidelinelines for Safe Surgery*. Geneva: World Health Organization.

World Health Organization. (2009). *Child growth standards and the identification of severe acute malnutrition in infants*. Geneva: WHO.

Resources

The Sphere Handbook | Standards for quality humanitarian response (sphere-standards.org)

www.healthservicecorps.org/training

https://www.who.int/nutrition/publications/severemalnutrition/9789241598163/en/

Chapter 3
Evidence-based Patient Safety-centered Culture

"To err is human; to cover up is unforgivable; and to fail to learn is inexcusable."

Sir Liam Donaldson

Best Practice Guideline 1
Build a Patient Safety Centered Organizational Culture

1.1. Create a patient safety and healthcare quality policy

1.2. Make the patient safety and healthcare quality policy publicly available

1.3. Include patient safety in organizational board meetings and project planning meetings

1.4. Designate a patient safety officer

Best Practice Guideline 1
Build a Patient Safety-centered Organizational Culture

The first guideline is to create a patient safety culture, and it is directed primarily toward the leadership of organizations that engage in global health care projects. This includes churches, universities, and any organizations that send healthcare providers to serve as volunteers in global health. It is important that all volunteers and project leaders keep building a culture of patient safety at the core of their work, if it involves healthcare delivery. This is also true for long-term global health workers, who are often practicing in places that have had little exposure to patient safety concepts. But, what is a patient safety culture, and how can it be created within global health programs? According to the University of Manchester (2006), a patient safety culture is defined as one in which staff (or volunteers) have a constant and active awareness of the potential for things to go wrong. It is also a culture that is open and fair, and encourages people to speak up about mistakes (University of Manchester, 2006).

Leadership for quality and patient safety is challenging, because it requires building a culture that supports openness about mistakes. It requires casting a vision for the need, so the extra work required to assure patient safety can be justified by providers. This is especially challenging in global health because in many cultures around the world admitting mistakes is taboo. This makes building the openness that allows for honest discussion of errors extremely difficult. Leaders working cross-culturally in global health need to gain understanding of cultural and community development dynamics that will affect healthcare quality and patient safety. There are a couple leadership models and characteristics worth reviewing to assist us in improving healthcare quality in poor- and middle- income countries.

According to Reinertsen (2010), who wrote the chapter entitled "Leadership for Quality" in *The Healthcare Quality Book*, quality improvement is a manifestation of leadership based in humility. He identifies humility as an intrinsic characteristic of quality-promoting leadership. Leadership for healthcare quality in global health initiatives involves changing widely held assumptions and practices. This is because transformation in healthcare quality involves a radical process of reframing our values and beliefs in a way that transforms our systems and behaviors. Humility is essential in this process since transformation involves examining how we decide what is right and, when necessary, reshaping beliefs that underlie our value systems. This was written about health-delivery systems in North America, but it is even more relevant for global health leadership.

Humility is a crucial trait for working cross-culturally (especially for North Americans) because it is an intrinsic component of being able to admit our own deficiencies and our own need for change. We often exhibit thoughts, actions, and attitudes suggesting that we have all the answers and have come to fix all the problems. Steve Saint, a well-known missionary produced a two-set DVD series for training volunteers in the dynamics of cross-cultural work. It is called *Mission Dilemma,* and it is foundational training for any Christian global health volunteer, medical or nonmedical. In it, he interviews several "receivers" of North American missions, one of whom was Oscar Muriu, a Kenyan pastor who said, "Please don't come to fix us; we have been fixed so many times; we are a real mess now" (Muriu, 2006). He goes on to discuss how people from North America are problem solvers, which is a tremendous asset in some situations. However, when the North American with a "we can fix anything" attitude attempts to collaborate with people that have been trapped in systemic poverty, there is an unfortunate result. We often feel a sense of gratification and reward because we made a real "Mother Teresa" contribution to the world. The people on the receiving end are sometimes left feeling less intelligent, and less capable of meeting their own needs. This is one of the primary concerns about any type of cross cultural initiative. They make us feel good, but sometimes at the expense of the receivers feeling less able to accomplish goals for themselves. If we are not cognizant of our thoughts, actions, and attitudes, we can do much unintentional harm. Humility is an essential trait of global health leadership and for any volunteer working cross-culturally. We will discuss what it looks like to operate from humility in a later chapter. We will discuss specific tools that keep us centered in humility such as Participatory Learning and Action (PLA). If we lead volunteers or staff who serve in global health, tools such as PLA help us impart to them how to operate and lead from a place of humility.

The Institute for Healthcare Improvement (IHI) paper "Leadership Guide to Patient Safety" by Botwinick, Bosognano, and Haraden (2006) provides an effective leadership framework for quality improvement and patient safety in any healthcare program. The ideas they present are applicable to the leadership of any organization delivering healthcare services; this includes the leadership of both faith-based and humanitarian organizations. They also apply to both short-term volunteer medical team initiatives, and long-term cross-cultural healthcare work in hospitals and clinics.

Step one of the outlined processes is to "address strategic priorities, culture, and infrastructure," which is probably the most relevant step for global health organizations. The discussion of the processes will therefore concentrate on this section of the leadership guide and its relevant applications to global health initiatives. This step in the process is divided into five sub-steps: (a) establish patient safety as a strategic organizational priority, (b) assess organizational culture, (c) establish a culture supportive of patient safety, (d) address organizational infrastructure, and (e) learn about patient safety and methods for improvement (Botwinick et al., 2006).

The first, and most important priority for any global health program, is to accept the moral and ethical responsibility inherent to all healthcare delivery systems: to first do no harm. The next, is to elevate patient safety above the number of patients treated, the number of prescriptions given, and the number of volunteers deployed. Once these basic steps have been taken, the next step in the process is to assess program culture. They recommend many tools available through the IHI, the Institute of Medicine (IOM), and the World Health Organization (WHO) to assess safety culture within healthcare delivery programs. However, there is no one-size-fits-all questionnaire for this type of safety culture assessment in global health programs and organizations (Botwinick et al., 2006). The varying size and structure of global health programs and the infrastructure of the poor settings they often serve makes modification of these assessments necessary. The culture assessment process begins by looking at the program priorities and where patient safety is placed in those priorities.

Assessment of Safety Culture in Global Health Projects

If we are to create a patient safety culture in global health programs, the starting point is to assess our current status. Engaging in discussions about safety with staff and volunteers is a good place to begin assessing your present safety culture. Identifying core beliefs about the need for patient safety in the program, will also help determine whether change needs to occur and how it can be facilitated. In 2006, the University of Manchester published a series of patient safety culture assessments for healthcare delivery programs (University of Manchester, 2006). Their primary care paper is referenced multiple times in WHO patient safety documents, and is supported by the UK National Patient Safety Agency as the standard for assessing a patient safety culture. This framework defines nine dimensions of assessing a culture of safety within a healthcare delivery program. These dimensions appear, with some modification of the corresponding questions, to refine their application to cross-cultural healthcare delivery. The following questions will help you gauge where your program may need focused quality-improvement efforts. These questions are not meant to criticize any weaknesses in the patient safety procedures. They are meant to help every stakeholder contribute to improved patient safety for the projects and programs in which they serve. It should be a cooperative assessment with respondents from both the sending and receiving partners engaged in a global health partnership.

This table shows the nine dimensions of patient safety culture as defined by the University of Manchester Patient Safety Framework (MaPSaF) for Primary Care. The left side lists the dimensions, and the right side presents the way in which those dimensions are defined for global health programs. In some cultures, they may be very new ideas, and in many cultures, admitting mistakes, as mentioned earlier, is taboo. This makes western practices of mortality and morbidity rounds more difficult, and open discussion of mistakes difficult. Short-term involvement is unlikely to change deeply held cultural beliefs. However, beginning open dialog about mistakes and assessing our work can set an important example. This assessment tool, and others, can at least begin a discussion that could mold our organizational cultures towards improved patient safety. And over time, they can have the same effect on our receiving partners, as well as their facilities and health programs.

Table 1. Patient safety survey.

1. Commitment to quality	How much time is invested in developing the quality and safety agenda? Does your program have policies and procedures to maintain safety? What attempts are made to look beyond the organization for information about patient safety?
2. Priority given to patient safety	Do the organizational board meetings and/or project planning meetings include discussions on maintaining and improving patient safety? Where does responsibility lie for patient safety issues?
3. Perceptions of the cause of patient safety incidents	What sort of reporting systems are there? Are adverse events being monitored for in the community after your group leaves? If reports of adverse events occur, what is the plan to address them? If an adverse event were reported, would it be hidden or exposed to the community to learn from the event?
4. Investigation of patient safety incidents	How does your program monitor for adverse events? Who investigates incidents, and how are they investigated? Is the documentation of your providers meeting international standards for healthcare delivery, and is it being evaluated?
5. Organizational learning following patient-safety incidents	If you have had a known incident, what happens after the incident? What mechanisms are in place to learn from the incident? How are changes introduced and evaluated?
6. Communication about safety issues	Are volunteers and staff oriented about patient safety? If so, how much training do they receive? Is there cultural orientation related to healthcare delivery for volunteers? Are volunteers trained in global health competencies and managing areas, such as childhood malnutrition and tropical disease?

7. Personnel management and safety issues	How are safety issues managed in the field? Are emergency anaphylaxis medications available, and is there staff trained in their use? Are there protocols for managing adverse medication events? How does staff and volunteer selection occur, and are volunteers willing to submit to safety orientation?
8. Staff education and training about safety issues	How, why, and when are education and training programs on patient safety developed? What do staff and volunteers think of them?
9. Teamwork around safety issues	How much teamwork is there around patient-safety issues? Is there a patient-safety officer (PSO) for the organization? Are sites selected to sustain patient safety? Is patient flow at field sites designed around patient safety or something else?

The MaPSaF also defines five levels of patient safety culture maturity: (a) pathological, (b) reactive, (c) bureaucratic, (d) proactive, and (e) generative. The lowest level, a pathologic culture, reflects the following characteristics: (a) information is often hidden, (b) messengers are "shot," (c) responsibilities are shirked, (d) bridging is discouraged, (e) failure is covered up, and (f) safety-promoting ideas are often crushed. The highest level all programs should aspire to achieve, a generative patient-safety culture, has the following characteristics: (a) messengers are trained, not shot; (b) responsibilities for safety are shared; (c) bridging to improve safety is rewarded; (d) patient-safety failure causes inquiry, not cover-up; and (e) new ideas to improve safety are welcomed (University of Manchester, 2006).

Table 2. Patient-safety framework for primary care
(Source: University of Manchester, 2006).

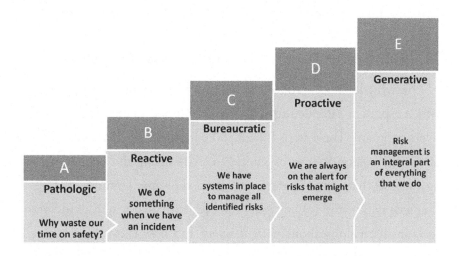

If your global health projects are like most, after reading through the previous questions, you will grade yourself closer to a pathologic patient safety culture than a generative one. The sad reality is many hospitals and clinics in resource poor communities fall into this pathologic category also. Poor attention to patient safety, by visiting healthcare professionals from wealthy countries, can reinforce pathologic healthcare safety cultures. I would argue the reverse is also true. Focused attention to patient safety may have some influence on the receiving facility culture.

Developing an effective cross-cultural medical or surgical outreach is a complex undertaking. It is believed by many that adding patient safety policies and procedures can make facilitating a complex project even more difficult. However, this not necessarily the case if programs have some basic guidelines to follow, like the ones found in this book. The end goal for any healthcare delivery program is not just to be aware of patient safety, but to reach a generative approach to patient safety in healthcare delivery. The ultimate goal, perhaps, being to bring our receiving national partners with us on this journey toward generative patient safety cultures.

1.1. Create a patient safety and healthcare quality policy.

Botwinick et al. (2006) outline some functional steps through which a patient safety culture can be established in any healthcare delivery program. These steps include (a) educating the board of directors about the responsibility for safety; (b) structuring the board meeting agendas so that patient safety is allotted the same amount of time as financial issues; and (c) engaging the executive board, staff, and volunteers in discussions about patient safety and how it can be improved. This may look different depending on whether it is a church mission team supervised by a mission board, a para-church mission organization communicating with a board of directors, or a university engaging in global health, but the concept is the same. Educating on the responsibility for patient safety is a good place to begin, since most boards see global health initiatives as charity work. They often do not realize the significant potential for harm inherent in healthcare delivery. One of the easiest ways to educate board members, staff, and volunteers, is to have a clearly defined policy around patient safety. Then, of course, make sure that policy is communicated and used as a tool for education.

1.2. Make the patient safety policy publicly available.

Organizations, such as Smile Train and Operation Smile, provide good examples of this type of public statement of their commitment to healthcare quality and patient safety (Medical Professionals Smile Train Safety Protocols, 2009; Operation Smile Global Standards of Care, 2011). Making patient safety policy publicly available on the organization's website, and in other ways, can help hold the organization accountable to living it out.

1.3. Include Patient Safety in organizational board meetings and project-planning meetings

Assessing minutes from the last four organizational board meetings, looking for discussions of safety, is a good beginning point in evaluating the culture of a global health program's commitment to patient safety (Botwinick et al. 2006). Reviewing meetings can provide a good snapshot of the present safety culture. If it is a church, university, or other organization that sends medical groups as a small part of their organizational mission, then this would apply to project planning meetings. The leaders of larger organizations (such as universities or churches) sending groups as one small part of their activities, need to understand that their organization is accepting the responsibility and liability for healthcare delivery.

As a side note, International Helpers (Guernsey Trust) is the only international malpractice insurance available at present. Each provider and organization needs to weigh the risks and decide if such insurance is needed. It is highly recommended for short-term anesthesia and surgical providers.

1.4. Designate a patient safety officer (PSO)

Botwinick et al. (2006) recommend that one person be in charge of patient safety for the organization, a PSO, and that the PSO report directly to the executive-level officers of the organization. They describe the PSO as having responsibility and accountability for driving a culture of safety within the organization. That person is responsible for designing, monitoring, and evaluating safety and quality improvement programs (Botwinick et al., 2006). There is clear application to volunteer medical and global health programs in this recommendation; designating a PSO role as a position of authority will help hold the program accountable to change.

The PSO model is also highly recommended in *The Healthcare Quality Book* chapter entitled "Organizational Quality Infrastructure" (Al-Assaf, 2008). Al-Assaf affirms the concept of one person having accountability to the organizational CEO (or program leadership) for quality assurance (QA), quality control (QC), and quality improvement (QI), all of which are part of a total quality management program. Al-Assaf (2008) also defines healthcare quality management as a cycle that requires two primary components: senior management support and a healthcare quality coordinator or PSO. The PSO's job is to drive improvement through a ten-step cycle, which includes (a) planning and reassessing, (b) setting standards, (c) communicating standards, (d) monitoring improvement initiatives, (e) identifying and prioritizing areas in need of improvement, (f) defining what QI should look like within their specific organizational context, (g) identifying who will work on QI teams and committees, (h) analyzing and studying QI initiatives, (i) choosing and designing solutions, and (j) implementing solutions (Al-Assaf, 2008).

The ideal person for a PSO position may not be available in a volunteer-driven global health organization, but a person having a willingness to read and learn about methods would be a minimum. Optimally, the PSO should have an understanding of, or a willingness to learn about, healthcare-specific QI-implementation models such as PDSA (Plan Do Study Act) and Rapid Cycle Testing, which is an IHI model designed to implement quality improvement initiatives in as short a time period as possible (Warren, 2008). In global healthcare programs, this position can be filled by a full-time paid person or a healthcare professional willing to volunteer his or her time in pursuit of patient safety. A registered nurse often holds this position in domestic health systems and may be an excellent selection for this position within global health organizations. This position should also be advocated for by long-term workers in the hospitals and health programs where they serve.

References

Al-Assaf, A. (2008). Organizational quality infrastructure: How does an organization staff quality? In E. R. Ranson, M. S. Joshi, D. B. Nash, & S. B. Ransom (Eds.), *The healthcare quality book: Vision, strategy and tools* (2nd ed., pp. 331-348). Chicago/Washington, DC: Health Administration Press.

Botwinick, L., Bosognano, M., & Haraden, C. (2006). *A leadership guide to patient safety.* Cambridge: Institute for Healthcare Improvement.

Medical Professionals Smile Train Safety Protocols. (2009). *Smile train.* Retrieved from http://medpro.smiletrain.org/medpro/safety/safetyprotocol.htm

Muriu, O. (2006, January). Pastor of Nairobi Chapel. (S. Saint, Interviewer)

Operation Smile Global Standards of Care. (2011). *Operation Smile.* Retrieved from http://www.operationsmile.org/our_work/global-standards-of-care/

Reinertsen, J. L. (2010). Leadership for quality. In E. R. Ransom, M. S. Joshi, D. B. Nash, & S. B. Ransom (Eds.), *The healthcare quality book* (pp. 311-328). Washington, DC: Health Administration Press.

University of Manchester. (2006). *The Manchester patient safety framework for primary care.* Manchester, UK: University of Manchester.

Warren, K. (2008). Quality improvement: The foundation, processes, tools, and knowledge transfer techniques. In E. R. Ransom, J. S. Maulik, D. B. Nash, & S. B. Ransom (Eds.), *The healthcare quality book* (2nd ed., pp. 63-83). Chicago/Washington, DC: Health Administration Press/AUPHA Press.

Chapter 4
Go as Learner not as Teacher

"He has shown you, O man, what is good; And what does the LORD require of you But to do justly, To love mercy, And to walk humbly with your God?"

- The Old Testament Profit Micah

Best Practice Guideline 2
Go as Learner not as Teacher

2.1. Recognize you have a lot to learn

2.2. Learn something about medication safety

2.3. Learn something about culture

2.4. Learn something about global health

2.5. Learn something about community health education

2.1. Recognize you have a lot to learn

Best Practice Guideline 1 reflects a need for anyone engaged in global health work to understand the potential harm that can result from not keeping patient safety at the center of their efforts. But it is also important to recognize that as healthcare professionals trained in wealthy countries, we are not prepared to practice in a resource-poor hospital or clinic. Since there is so much we do not know, we have to approach this work as a learner — not as a teacher. We must step into this context with great humility with a genuine desire to learn what our national colleagues and long-term workers have to teach us.

I must admit that short-term medical volunteers that come to support our staff at hospitals are far less helpful than we would hope. Partly because they are functioning in a new environment, but mainly because they are not prepared. We do not see children critically ill with severe acute malnutrition, cerebral malaria, dengue, or TB while practicing in a wealthy country. This is an enormous learning curve for anyone, especially those serving for a short time. Few healthcare professionals keep up with global health research. For example, the Feast study done in 2010 found that our typical fluid bolus strategy for children with sepsis was harmful to children in Africa. The study had to be stopped early because they found boluses significantly increased 48-hour mortality in critically ill children in Africa. Essentially, our normal standard of practice for septic children in wealthy countries has been shown to cause the death of some African children (Maitland, et al., 2011) .

It's not just medical practice that is very different in resource-poor settings. Surgical practice is also very different. Surgeons who work in global health are often required to manage a much wider range of patients. Often, when a surgeon reaches out to our organization to work full-time overseas, they want to teach surgery in Africa. I am excited for them but try to help them see they probably need to learn how to do surgery in Africa before they can teach it. General surgeons in bush hospitals are often required to do a lot of orthopedic work, burns, neurosurgery, pediatric surgery, and OB/GYN etc. General surgeons often have to manage all the subspecialty areas of surgery they would normally not care for in their home country. It's also true that most bush hospitals do not have laparoscopic surgical capabilities, making every surgery and open case.

It should be said however, that going as a learner means we learn all we can before going to serve in a resource poor-setting. We can look to our national colleagues and long-term global medical workers to teach us a lot. However, pre-field preparation is also important. It's hard for someone to teach us the 10-step protocol for treating a child with severe acute malnutrition if we have never even seen the protocol. Whether we are planning to serve long-term or short-term, there is a place for pre-field preparation. Existing practice guidelines for re-source-poor settings and patient safety should be the primary focus of pre-field learning.

"Standards of Excellence for Short-term Missions" describes pre-field training as one of seven standards to which programs should ad-here (Collins, 2006). However, in short-term global health programs, pre-field orientation on patient safety is a minimum requirement—not a standard of excellence. Patient safety issues may vary depending on the type of healthcare program, but there are some areas of knowledge with which all volunteers need to be familiar. These general patient safety issues include pharmacovigilance, regional cultural beliefs about healthcare and medications, and global health core competencies. It's incumbent on providers to learn a little about each of these areas before stepping into a resource-poor context.

2.2. Learn about medication safety - pharmacovigilance

No medication is without risk, and the risk versus benefit of medications needs to be carefully assessed by every prescriber. Training for healthcare providers on prescribing in resource-poor settings is a fundamental responsibility of sending programs. According to the World Health Organization (2006), pharmacovigilance refers to the science and activities relating to the detection, assessment, understanding, and prevention of adverse events or any possible medication-related problems. Pharmacovigilance programs at the national policy level involve comprehensive surveillance and reporting of adverse drug events over the lifecycle of a medication to improve safety. However, every health program has the responsibility to develop policies and procedures that promote safer prescribing, dispensing, and administration practices. It is incumbent on global health programs to develop a pharmacovigilance program and to communicate related policies and procedures to their staff and volunteers. These policies should be developed on a sound evidence base and follow all relevant WHO dispensing guidelines and home country practices, which are outlined in detail under Best Practice Guideline 3. The pharmacovigilance policy should be part of the patient safety policy described in the previous chapter.

2.3. Learn something about culture

Cross-cultural healthcare competence training is a minimum standard strongly supported literature. Betancourt, Green, and Carrillo define cultural competence in healthcare as "the ability of providers and systems to provide care to patients with diverse values, beliefs, and behaviors, including tailoring delivery to meet patients' social, cultural, and linguistic needs" (2002). This is a challenging but appropriate definition for global health initiatives. It is the responsibility of medical sending and/or receiving programs to educate their volunteers about cultural beliefs and practices that affect how medications and healthcare are perceived by the local population.

According to the WHO document "Patient Safety in African Health Services: Issues and Solutions" (2008), more than half of all patients fail to take prescribed medications properly. They also report that in African countries, high levels of illiteracy combined with cultural and societal beliefs about medications and healthcare drastically affect patient safety in negative ways (WHO, 2008). The frequency of medications being shared in the community, culturally conditioned assumptions (e.g., injections have mystical power, pill colors or size determining purpose), and propensity to share medications, are all important for providers to understand. Knowing medications dispensed may be sold or traded for other items is also important. Education on these topics can assist volunteer healthcare providers in making culturally appropriate modifications to the care they render to patients. This kind of cultural training is essential for global health initiatives.

According to Betancourt, Weissman, Kim, Park, and Maina (2007), few physicians in the US have had formal training on cross-cultural communication and care, and many do not feel prepared to provide care cross-culturally. Treating patients whose worldview conflicts with western medicine is a specific concern. According to Transcultural Nursing Society (2010), organizations need to provide ongoing educational workshops as well as mentoring and training geared toward the continuous development of nurses' cultural knowledge and skills for effective cross-cultural practice. If this regionally-specific cultural competence training is not provided by the facilitating organization, it is the professional responsibility of providers to learn all they can about healthcare provision in the country and region in which they will be serving.

2.4. Learn something about global health

It is considered a minimum standard that international medical programs provide information on core global health competencies required for safe practice in resource-poor countries. This book is a good starting place to understand core global health competencies. The extent of preparation needed depends on the planned duration of service. For those planning to serve as a healthcare professional in a short- or long-term capacity, here are some recommendations. The depth of study may vary with duration of service.

Tropical Medicine – diagnosis and treatment of tropical pathologies such as malaria, dengue fever, TB, leprosy, etc.

IMCI – Integrated Management of Childhood Illness

IMAM – Integrated Management of Acute Malnutrition

IMPCB – Integrated Management of Pregnancy and Childbirth

WHO Safe Surgery Program and Checklist

We will discuss some of these in later chapters, and you can find out more about these programs on the CHSC clinical resource page at https://www.healthservicecorps.org/clinical_resources/. We have compiled a good number of global health self-study resources on this page you may find helpful. In addition to WHO resources, you will also find links to the Johns Hopkins School of Public Health open-source learning modules in international healthcare, and the USAID Global Health Learning Center. I would recommend both of these open-source e-learning centers for free online training in global health competencies. For those looking for in-person or virtual classroom courses, I would recommend any of the Christian Health Service Corps continuing education courses. They include Global Health and Tropical Medicine Overview, Disaster and Refugee Response (sphere training), Community Health Evangelism, and Teaching Healthcare in the Global Setting (our faculty development course). Although, CHSC is a faith-based organization and the courses do include some faith orientation, everyone is welcome, but the faith orientation may be uncomfortable for some participants. https://www.healthservicecorps.org/

The Institute for International Medicine (INMED) offers mixed online and in person diploma courses in international healthcare with several opportunities for overseas healthcare internships around the world. They have also begun offering a master's degree in international health. https://www.inmed.us/

2.5. Learn something about community health education

The need for community health education in low- and middle- income countries cannot be overstated. In many communities, the prevalence of problems such as pediatric/infant mortality, and maternal mortality are alarmingly high. Health education interventions have proven effective in addressing many of the causes of child mortality. For example, studies show that better breastfeeding practices alone could save 800,000 lives per year (Vesel et al., 2009). Micronutrient supplementation has been shown to have a notable positive impact on the long-term development and reduction in mortality of malnourished children in developing communities. According to Vesel et al. (2009), Vitamin A supplementation can reduce mortality by up to 23%. Another study (Imdad, et al., 2011) looked at 21 different studies on the effectiveness of Vitamin A supplementation and found similar results. They showed a 25% reduction in child mortality from all causes and a 30% reduction related to diarrheal illnesses.

Iron supplementation has also been shown to impact child development over age two, and zinc supplementation has been shown to reduce diarrhea incidence by 18% and pneumonia incidence by 41% (Vesel et al., 2009). The present WHO recommendations are that Vitamin A supplementation programs work alongside health promotion and communication activities (Hill, Kirkwood, & Edmond, 2004).

Although these studies seem old, research continues to validate these interventions as effective in reducing under 5 mortalities in low- and middle-income countries (LMIC's). This is especially true in encouraging exclusive breastfeeding practices. A 2018 UNICEF report reaffirmed that exclusive breastfeeding practices could save the lives of an estimated 820,000 children annually (UNICEF, 2018).

The WHO recommends four general health education interventions that have been proven to reduce child mortality. These are also found in the IMCI Chart Booklet. It is highly recommended that caregivers of children receive counseling on at least one of these health education areas each time they visit a clinic. Global providers should be prepared to counsel on all of these areas within the cultural context of the community they will be serving.

1. Care-seeking behaviors of parents (when to seek care)

2. Nutrition (maternal and child)

3. Home management of diarrhea and dehydration

4. Malaria prevention, where appropriate (maternal and child)

(WHO/UNICEF, 2014)

The IMCI Chart Booklet provides specific breastfeeding assessment and counseling instructions. Along with dosing for vitamin A, iron, and zinc supplementation for children in low- and middle-income countries (LMIC's) (WHO/UNICEF, 2014). You can download a copy of the IMCI Chart Booklet from the Christian Health Service Corps website on the clinical resources page.

"Short-term Medical Teams – What They Do Well... and Not So Well,"

Dohn and Dohn, their 2006 "Short-term Teams – What They Do Well . . . and Not So Well," describe health education as one area that medical groups do "not so well." This is primarily because short-term volunteers attempt to provide such education through translators and with inadequate cultural and worldview understanding. When we, from a different culture, attempt to engage in education without first learning about the context and developing a relationship, there is always the potential for less than favorable outcomes. Cross-cultural health education is challenging because we are faced with what many in low- and middle-income countries refer to as the "God complex dilemma." This idea was first presented to me many years ago at a week-long workshop given by Jaisankar Sarma, a longtime community development practitioner and former head of International Development at World Vision. As a native of India, he shared how westerners are often seen from the perspective of the poor and how our subconscious and subliminal attitudes can drastically affect our interactions with the poor. He shared that poverty is, to a large extent, a manifestation of a marred identity and self-worth. Without adequate understanding, volunteers from developed countries leading health education classes in developing countries can further mar the identity of those they seek to serve. We need to engage in such activities with extreme caution, sensitivity, and humility, knowing as much about the culture, worldview, and life circumstances as possible.

The two pictures below illustrate two very different methods of approaching local communities. In the first picture, the health worker is standing in front dispensing information to the local people. The people are expected to sit and listen as though they are children. In the second picture, the health worker is sitting down and having a conversation with them. They are able to interact as equals who can share information and ideas and learn from each other.

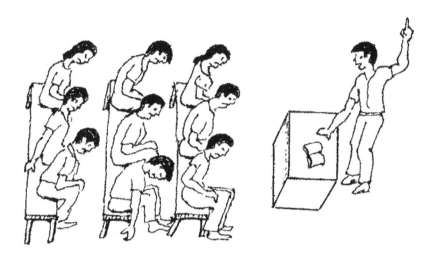

Health education <u>should not</u> look like this.

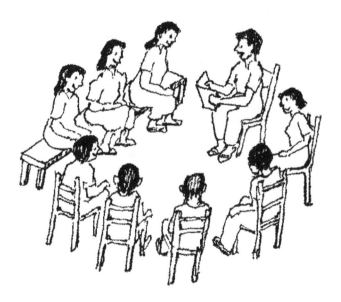

Health education <u>should</u> look like this.

There is more to be caught than to be taught

Learning something about cross-cultural health education in the area is good practice for volunteer clinicians because we must educate our patients as we care for them. Physicians, nurses, and pharmacists provide health education and counseling on health topics as part of our patient consultations. But as a rule, health education for groups in a community is best done by people who share the same cultural context—mostly because it is very hard to cross the cultural divide on health. And it goes beyond culture. People volunteering in low- and middle- income countries are operating from the top of Maslow's Pyramid. We are meeting higher developmental needs of contribution, meaning, and purpose. In short, we are usually operating from the self-actualization end of the pyramid. The people being served are usually operating from the bottom of that pyramid, trying to meet basic survival needs. This itself is an enormous cultural barrier.

If we seek to help people make changes in their own health, it is important to understand that poor health is often part of a cycle created by poverty. Poverty, as a manifestation of a marred identity, shapes people's collective worldview. Worldview is the lens through which people view their world. Stated another way, it is the roots that underlie all belief systems and behavioral patterns. The intertwined complexities of values, cultural norms, individual and collective self-worth, gender inequities, education, crop choices, food choices, and beliefs about health are all driven by worldview. For example, in some West African communities, children are not fed meat or protein. It is believed it will cause them to become delinquents or thieves. Such practices result in extremely high levels of protein-energy malnutrition, correlating to equally high pediatric mortality. When dealing with such issues, exercise caution. Succumbing to the temptation to tell people that their culturally formed traditions and practices are wrong or foolish will not result in the desired change. Even if they want to see changes that will result in better health and a better quality of life, generations of traditions and taboos as well as pressure from within the community make it nearly impossible. The inability of individuals within the society to make these changes can further mar the identity of a struggling young mother when she is given instructions by a foreigner that she is unable to carry out.

About 70% of people around the world live in collectivist societies. Among other things, this means that the community must decide as a group to make changes for transformation to occur. Community leaders including government officials, pastors, elders, and other respected members of the society are often key stakeholders in decisions about proper behavior within the community—even those related to health—which westerners would consider to be personal decisions. Discussion and building relationships are important places to begin. Although change tends to be a slow process, the advantage of working with collectivist societies is that each individual within the society does not need to be convinced about the benefits of changes in their health practices or beliefs. If the community decides to make changes, everyone will be encouraged to make these changes together. Changing behavior in this context requires changing the underlying worldview of the entire community. This requires long-term commitment and living among the poor. A complete change will not occur as a result of any one group visiting a community, but such challenges represent an exceptional opportunity to serve and support the efforts of local partners. Lingenfelter and Mayers' book *Ministering Cross-Culturally: A Model for Effective Relationships* (2016) was written with Christians doing cross cultural work in mind. However, it provides an exceptional discussion on developing cross-cultural partnerships for any reader. It helps in processing through tensions in the areas of time, judgment, handling crises, goals, self-worth, and vulnerability.

It is also important to remember that health education is only successful in the context of a facilitative model. Facilitators inspire change at the deepest levels by asking questions that reveal the roots of the problems. Change occurs only when the community discovers the roots of its problems and develops its own processes of responding to them. It is best to consider this in the context of assisting and supporting community partners to effect lasting change.

One of the most valuable tools we have found for training health educators is to have them assume the responsibilities of a young mother in a poor community for a few days. Once they have lived, eaten, and slept in the community as well as carried the burden of a young mother, they are much better qualified to speak into her life. Before educators can speak to a young mother, telling her she must boil all water for drinking and other such tasks, they must understand how hard her life already is and what they are adding to it. Once they assume the responsibilities of caring for children, making food from scratch over an open fire, collecting wood, sometimes making charcoal, washing clothes in the river, and bathing in the river, they soon realize that health education is more complex than they thought. They need to help mothers develop strategies to meet the health needs of their families in the context of their incredibly difficult lives. We need to listen and observe and not try to impose our solutions, because the average volunteer has no understanding of the life context into which they are attempting to speak. Listen, observe, learn, and share the vital information and aspects of health. There is an old community development saying that goes, "There is more to be caught than to be taught."

Sharing our lives with local people and demonstrating positive health practices will go further to help people understand what change could look like than any lecture. The ideal health education program is the Community Health Empowerment (CHE) model where the focus is on training community educators—not the general population in the community. Volunteers then serve and support the work and efforts of those educators. Many international groups that include health education as part of each patient encounter do this and do not even realize it. By the end of a one- or two-week community project, their translators are experienced educators for the community. However, it is better to accomplish this using a more intentional approach rather than hoping it will happen by accident. In the next chapter, we present an example of how we have used the method of health education by local educators in combination with healthcare teams.

Resources

There are many health education programs and curriculums available. Health Education Programs for Developing Countries is the resource I recommend the most since it is evidence based, free, and is best suited for counseling patients in exam rooms. Health Books International (formerly TALC - Teaching Aids at Low Cost) is a UK-based program that has other important training materials for volunteers and for the community. The Global CHE network is an excellent resource for learning how to design Christian community health programs that will train local health educators. The Hesperian Foundation also has a wide range of resources available for community-based programs. They are also an excellent resource for groups that would like to help the community create their own health education materials. They now make all of the Hesperian publication illustrations available for download online along with templates for creating posters and brochures.

We highly recommend that global projects evaluate these resources and make the Hesperian resources and their website known to coworkers in low- and middle- income countries. Their resources are available in many languages, and because of their vast image library, the resources are adaptable to various local cultures. In later chapters we will look at how these ideas fold into the community empowerment and building capacity. Here is a list of resources you may find helpful.

Resources Listed for Global Health Training

Christian Health Service Corps www.healthservicecorps.org (under resources and courses)

Community Toolbox http://ctb.ku.edu/en/default.aspx

Global CHE Network http://chenetwork.org/

Global Health eLearning Center sponsored by USAID http://www.globalhealthlearning.org/

Health Education Program for Developing Countries www.hepfdc.info

Hesperian Health Guides http://hesperian.org/books-and-resources/

INMED - the Institute for International Medicine https://www.inmed.us/

Medicus Mundi of Switzerland www.healthtraining.org

Mother and Child Nutrition Protocols http://motherchildnutrition.org/

Health Books International https://healthbooksinternational.org/

See Appendix for a comprehensive resource list of WHO global health materials

References

Betancourt, J. R., Green, A. R., & Carrillo, J. E. (2002). *Cultural competence in healthcare: Emerging frameworks and practical approaches.* New York: The Commonwealth Fund.

Betancourt, J. R., Weissman, J. S., Kim, M. K., Park, E. R., & Maina, A. W. (2007). *Resident physicians' preparedness to provide cross-cultural care: Implications for clinical care and medical education policy.* New York: The Commonwealth Fund.

Collins, J. (2006). Standards of excellence in short-term missions. *Common Ground Journal,* 10-16.

Dohn, M. N., & Dohn , A. L. (2003). Quality of care on short term medical missions: experience with a standardized medical record and related issues. *Missiology: An International Review* , 417-429.

Global Health Education Consortium. (2011). GHEC homepage. *Global Health Education.* Retrieved from http://globalhealtheducation.org/SitePages/Home.aspx

Hill, Z., Kirkwood, B., & Edmond, K. (2004). *Family and community practices that promote child survival,growth and development A REVIEW OF THE EVIDENCE.* Geneva: World Health Organization .Transcultural Nursing Society. (2010, December 30). Standards of practice for cultural competence. *Transcultural Nursing Society.* Retrieved from http://www.tcns.org/TCNStandardsofPractice.html

Imdad, A., Yakoob, M. Y., Sudfeld, C., Haider, B. A., Black, R. E., & Bhutta, Z. A. (2011). Impact of vitamin A supplementation on infant and childhood mortality. *BMC Public Health.* Retrieved from https://bmcpublichealth.biomedcentral.com/articles/10.1186/1471-2458-11-S3-S20

Transcultural Nursing Society. (2010, December 30). *Standards of Practice for Cultural Competence* . Retrieved October 30th, 2011, from Transcultural Nursing Society: http://www.tcns.org/TCNStandardsofPractice.html

Vesel, L., Bahl, R., Martines, J., Penny, M., Bhandari, N., & Groupe, B. K.-l. (2009). Infant malnutrition assessed using new WHO child growth standards and its relationship with mortality and exclusive breastfeeding. *Publication: Bulletin of the World Health Organization; Type: Research* .

WHO/UNICEF. (2005). *IMCI Handbook.* Geneva: WHO Press.

WHO . (2006). The safety of medications in public health programmes:Pharmacovigilance as an essential tool. Geneva: WHO .World Health Organization. (2008). *Patient safety in African health services: Issues and solutions.* Yaounde, Republic of Cameroon: WHO Regional Committee for Africa.

Chapter 5
First Do No Harm

5.1. Stay within scope of practice

5.2. Practice pharmacovigilance

Best Practice Guideline 3 - Practice Patient Safety

Best Practice Guideline 1 speaks to developing a culture of patient safety and the steps necessary to facilitate this within our organizations. Guideline 3–Practice Patient Safety looks at how we implement patient safety processes in cross-cultural healthcare delivery. Developing patient safety systems for global medical programs is a matter of maintaining all safety processes normally followed in the volunteer provider's home country. Specific methods and processes of patient flow and logistical operations are open to collaboration and mutual design. However, those evidence-based performance measures practiced in the provider's home country or set forth by WHO must be followed. The guidelines listed here are about centering clinic flow and patient care on patient safety principles. Many programs orient the clinic flow around community health education, general efficiency, and even evangelism with Christian projects. The primary point in the development of Best Practice Guideline 3 is that safety comes first in projects that involve healthcare delivery. Patient safety is best achieved by following clinical practice guidelines, clinical pathways, and other evidence-based recommendations.

5.1. Practice only within scope of practice

Maintaining scope of practice is a basic standard for practicing in all countries. Would a radiologist see and treat a patient as a primary care physician in his/her home country? Would an OB/GYN provide primary healthcare to pediatric patients in his/her home country? Would a floor nurse prescribe medications in his/her home country? Of course not, yet we see these role transitions frequently when medical volunteers take part in global medical projects that serve the poor. These types of role transitions clearly do not support patient safety. Practicing outside normal scope of practice is common in volunteer projects that provide medical care in village communities. At the heart of going outside one's scope of practice is the common volunteer assumption discussed earlier (i.e., "Something is better than nothing."). However, we must seriously question that rationale when the something has the potential to cause harm. Allowing volunteers or students to operate outside their normal scope of practice can be harmful. But it also lacks a fundamental respect for the people being served. The overriding practice standard in all global health projects is simple: any and all patient safety and regulatory standards that a provider is subject to in his or her home country apply everywhere. Safety standards do not have international boundaries. If one would not, should not, or could not do it for a patient in one's home country, one should not do it when providing care as part of a global healthcare initiative. Healthcare volunteers and global health service-learning students are also governed under this best practice guideline. Whatever their specific level of training allows them to do in their home country with that level of supervision is what they can do during volunteer service.

Another issue that often presents itself is permission to practice. We must obtain permission to practice for each volunteer healthcare professional. It is the law in all countries, so appropriate channels must be followed to obtain permission to practice. The specific professions that require permission vary from country to country, as do the procedures. The International Association of Medical Regulatory Authorities (see http://www.iamra.com/) has some credentialing resources listed by country. Partnering permanent healthcare facilities are likely aware of the process to obtain a temporary professional license if needed. Non-healthcare partners are rarely aware of these processes and procedures.

5.2 Practice pharmacovigilance

If you question the rationale for these standards, remember that more than half of all medications are prescribed, dispensed, or sold inappropriately, and half of all patients fail to take medicines correctly (WHO, 2010). It is no surprise then that most of the patient safety concerns with community-based healthcare programs revolve around medication usage and dispensing practices. Pharmacovigilance policies may vary according to respective organization strategy and type of group (e.g., university service learning, medical, surgical, dental, health education or all the above). However, all policies need to reflect WHO safety standards and guidelines and the safety practices volunteer providers use in their home country. There are many standards that apply to all volunteers in global health. It is also important to note the WHO makes no distinction between safety practices in wealthy versus low- and middle-income countries. Examples of medication safety standards that need to be met by all healthcare providers include dispensing all potentially toxic medications in child-resistant containers (Poison Prevention Packaging Act [PPPA], 1970, as cited in The Consumer Product Safety Commission, 2005). They are inexpensive and weigh very little, making their transport with the visiting providers easy to accomplish. A list of places to purchase child-resistant containers can be acquired by searching for pharmacy supplies on the internet. Other such standards set by the WHO include giving patient instructions in closed, private consultation rooms free of distractions—not at open pharmacy counters in front of a crowd of people. The WHO also requires caregivers receiving medications for small children to verbally explain the dosing procedure and demonstrate the administration of the first dose to the child (WHO/UNICEF, 2005). These are minimum standards established by the WHO for the protection of children and families in all countries. We follow these standards in wealthy countries without question. They are especially important in poor communities. This is because safe storage of medications is a serious challenge when the family home is a one-room, dirt floor shelter.

According to the WHO (2008), approximately 125 children per day lose their lives because of poisonings—the vast majority of which are pharmaceutical-related. One study from the United Arab Emirates found that 55% of childhood poisonings were medication-related, with analgesics, non-steroidal anti-inflammatory drugs (NSAIDs), and antihistamines being the most common causes in the one-to-five-year age group. Another study from Turkey also showed that accidental ingestion of medications was the most common cause of poisoning in children aged one to five years at 57.7%. This same study also confirmed the most frequent medications were analgesics and NSAIDs. Yet another study from Bangladesh, Colombia, Egypt, and Pakistan showed medications were responsible for 31% of poisonings in children under 12 years of age (WHO, 2008).

It is also important to note that prior to the 1970 PPPA, child poisonings were largely considered the leading cause of death in children aged one to five in the U.S., with pharmaceuticals as the leading poisons (The Consumer Product Safety Commission, 2005). These studies are highly suggestive that some specific medications such as NSAIDs should be eliminated from the formularies of global health programs, and that dispensing medications in Ziploc plastic bags is neither safe nor appropriate. Ziploc baggies are never acceptable for dispensing pharmaceuticals.

Where volunteers serve and who is overseeing the project (volunteers or local providers) guides the program pharmacovigilance policies. It is worth noting, however, that many hospitals and health programs in low- and middle income countries do not have access to child-resistant containers and therefore use envelopes for dispensing some pills. Many pharmaceutical suppliers for low- and middle-income countries sell pills packaged in child resistant packets.

What we know about patient safety and quality assessment from the Donabedian theory tells us patient safety is difficult to achieve even within functional health systems.

Deciding what medications are safe in a village community should not be based solely on the WHO Model List of Essential Medicines. One assumption made by many global health and medical programs is that their medication formularies should be based on the WHO essential medicine list. If a short-term program is working in a permanent health system, this is a true and valid assumption. However, just because a medication is on the WHO list does not make it safe to use in every context. It is important to remember that all WHO materials and literature are directed at permanent health facilities not short-term community healthcare initiatives. The WHO Model List of Essential Medicines defines what medications should be available by respective country ministries of health in facilities they oversee (WHO, 2012). As of this writing in 2021, there are 574 medications on the WHO Model List of Essential Medicines —up from 276 when the first edition of this book was published in 2012.

Volunteers working in and under the direction of a permanent local health program may safely use many of the medications on the WHO Model List for Essential Medicines. Global medical projects operating in schools or churches apart from the local healthcare system could safely dispense only a small fraction of the WHO essential medicines. Most of them are not applicable for a rural clinic setting—in fact, there are only about 30 to 40 medications needed in a community clinic setting. Most rural health outposts in low- and middle-income countries function effectively with less than 20 medications. We will discuss some of them in more detail later.

The WHO document "Patient safety in African health services: Issues and solutions" (2008), also affirmed that more than half of all medications in Africa are prescribed, dispensed, or sold improperly, and more than half of the patients fail to take them properly. This report identifies that in African countries, this is most often a result of cultural and societal views. Cultural views of healthcare and medicines, when combined with high levels of illiteracy, pose significant barriers to patient safety (WHO, 2008). Formularies for global health should be focused on avoiding potential for adverse outcomes. If a global medical project is not directly connected to a permanent health program, limiting medications to acute pathologies treatable within the context of one clinic visit is strongly advisable. Treating chronic diseases without collaboration with local healthcare providers is neither safe nor appropriate. Global medical volunteer projects that treat chronic diseases (e.g., hypertension, chronic obstructive pulmonary disease, diabetes, epilepsy) require close collaboration with permanent health systems and should do so only from functional medical facilities and clinics.

Many of the medications on the Model List for Essential Medicines require continued patient monitoring. The list includes drugs for chemotherapy, palliative care, seizures, anticoagulation, and intravenous medications; contrast material, cardiac, contraceptive, serum/IGG, and obstetrical medications; as well as medications for TB, HIV, and leprosy. There is a growing body of evidence that supports significantly limiting prescriptions by volunteers from wealthy countries in global health projects. Focusing volunteers on prevention, health screening, and supporting regional public health efforts is far more helpful for chronic disease management. Donated medicines that require monitoring and ongoing follow-up should be given to local providers or long-term medical workers to dispense.

The following are basic evidence-based global health pharmacovigilance standards; each volunteer should review and understand these basic standards. Feel free to copy these items into your organization's patient safety policy.

5.2a. Prescribe medications only when absolutely necessary and <u>dispense them in child-resistant containers (not Ziploc plastic bags)</u>. Remember, there are no double standards for patient safety; standards that exist in developed countries also apply in developing countries. PPNN (a pill for every problem and a needle for every need) thinking should never be a part of global health initiatives for both patient safety and developmental reasons.

5.2b. Know the country's pharmaceutical dispensary laws and respect them. Ideally, a local pharmacist or team pharmacist should oversee the dispensing of medication. Unlicensed staff should never package, label, or dispense medication.

5.2c. No central pharmacy medication dispensing - This means that prescriptions may be filled in a central pharmacy area; however, medications should only be dispensed in the private consultation rooms or exam rooms. A licensed provider, pharmacist, or nurse may provide medication education and counseling. One-time dose medications (e.g., parasite prophylaxis, vitamin A supplementation) may be dispensed at a central location.

5.2d. Mothers or caretakers of children prescribed home medication must (for each child) verbalize the medication instructions, demonstrate measuring the dose of medication, and administer the first dose of the medication under the supervision of a licensed provider (nurse or physician). Again, this must happen in private pharmacy consultation rooms or exam rooms. Attempt to limit the number of prescriptions for each family. Each child treated should have medication dosages labeled with each child's name and age. Education before medication!

For community based medical programs, the system we have deployed to prevent overprescribing and to ensure the WHO standards are followed are simple. The healthcare provider must go to the pharmacy, get the medication, and come back and instruct the patient themself. Prior to leaving the clinic, the patient who receives medication is asked to explain the use of his or her medications to ensure full understanding. The educator then reinforces medication usage and provides information on one or two priority health education areas. To some, this sounds like it impedes patient flow; however, we have found it does not significantly decrease the number of patients seen. Even if it did, the improvements in patient safety would far outweigh any decrease in numbers. Remember, one of the central culprits in adverse outcomes in healthcare projects is prioritizing the number of patients seen over patient safety. It is better to treat one hundred patients well than a thousand patients and end up with a story like Maria's.

5.2e. Never take expired medications into a country. This is unlawful, and some countries have restrictions on the use of short dates. Know the country's standards. Some countries send a health inspector to the airport to ensure no medications coming in are less than 12 months from expiration.

5.2f. Never give samples or unlabeled medications unless it is a complete dosing regimen.

5.2g. Know and adhere to the WHO/UNICEF standards of practice in developing countries. We will discuss some of these later.

5.2h. Buy medications in-country when possible. If importing medications, create a detailed inventory of pharmaceuticals (with expiration dates). Leave medications in their original containers and never re-packaged for distribution prior to entering the country of service.

5.2i. Never leave surplus medications with unqualified healthcare personnel. If supplying medications to CHW programs, it is important to ensure adequate training on medications dispensing and the need for safe storage. Supplying medications for such programs comes with the responsibility of supplying child-resistant containers. Usually, families are instructed to keep such containers so they can be refilled with other medications and relabeled. Secure pharmaceuticals at all times, and patients must receive training on safe home storage to keep them away from children.

5.2j. Never attempt to sneak medications into a country. Think about what would happen to you if you were caught smuggling drugs into your home country. Pharmacy laws vary from country to country, but the least you can expect is for medications to be confiscated. In some countries, imprisonment is possible. Medications can often be purchased at very low costs in local pharmacies, and it is very helpful to develop relationships with local pharmacists.

In the next chapter we will discuss what medications are safe and needed in community clinics of low- and middle-income countries.

References

Chopra, M., Patel, S., Cloete, K., Sanders, D., & Peterson, S. (2005). Effect of an IMCI intervention on quality of care across four districts in Cape Town, South Africa. *Archives of Disease in Childhood, 90*, 397–401.

Luis, H., Robert, S., A Mwansa, N., & Cesa, R. V. (2008). How much does quality of care vary between health workers with different levels of training? An observational multi-country study. *The Lancet, Research Library Core, 372*, 910–916.

Tavrow, P., Rukyalekere, A., Maganda, A., Ndeezi, G., Sebina-Zziwa, A., & Knebel, E. (2002). *A comparison of computer-based and standard training in the integrated management of childhood illness in Uganda.* Bethesda: USAID by the Quality Assurance Project, University Research Co.

WHO Dept. of Child Health and Development. (2009, January). Child and adolescent health topics. Retrieved from http://www.who.int/child_adolescent_health/topics/prevention_care/child/imci/en/

WHO Secretary General. (2008). *Progress report on millennium development goals.* New York: United Nations Department of Economic and Social Affairs. Retrieved from http://www.un.org/millenniumgoals/pdf/The%20Millennium%20Development%20Goals%20Report%202008.pdf

Chapter 6
Big Picture Goals in Global Health

3.3. Use clinical practice guidelines for Community-based healthcare initiatives

"Pioneering spirit should continue, not to conquer the planet or
space ... but rather to improve the quality of life."

- Bertrand Piccard

3.3 Use clinical practice guidelines for Community-based healthcare initiatives

Following clinical practice guidelines and clinical pathways is
essential to safe practice in low- and middle-income countries
(LMICs). The challenge that many practitioners face is that
healthcare and medical practice look different in low- and middle-income countries. Many of the established treatment guidelines and protocols are unfamiliar to healthcare providers from resource-rich countries. There are standards for referral of one level of care to another,

and standards for classifying, diagnosing and treating diseases such as pneumonia based on clinical signs and symptoms—not X-rays. Patients often present with multiple pathologies, making accurate diagnosis challenging. Underlying malnutrition, endemic malaria, and so many other diseases of poverty can quickly put medical providers out of their depth. The World Health Organization has developed several clinical pathways and guidelines to assist providers. It is not possible for every global medical volunteer to learn every set of WHO guidelines; however, it is essential that the leadership of such programs have a working knowledge of such clinical guidelines. Before we discuss specific guidelines, it is worth looking at why and how many of these guidelines came into existence. They have driven a lot of progress in global health over the past three decades.

The Alma Ata Declaration

Best Practice Guideline 3 Practice Patient Safety discusses the importance of learning and following established clinical evidence-based guidelines set forth by the World Health Organization (WHO) and UNICEF. Before we can get there, we must first see such programs in the context in which they were designed. In order to follow clinical-practice guidelines for developing countries, we need to understand that their goals and objectives are often different. The thought process that created them is also different from our western (i.e., vertical) view of healthcare. In order to understand this thought process, we must look back to September of 1978. That year, an international convention took place known as the International Conference on Primary Health Care. It was developed by the two primary United Nations health agencies, WHO and UNICEF. It was attended by delegates from 134 governments, many international organizations, and many non-governmental organizations (NGOs). The NGOs present included both faith-based and strictly humanitarian charity programs.

The convention was held in Almaty Kazakhstan, which at that time was known as Kazakh Soviet Socialist Republic, part of the Soviet Union. The end result of the convention was a declaration known as the Declaration of Alma-Ata. This declaration called for urgent international action to develop and implement primary healthcare throughout the world, particularly in low- and middle-income countries. It urged governments, and the entire world community, to support the international commitment to primary healthcare. It also urged the channeling of technical and financial support to primary healthcare, specifically in low- and middle-income countries. The declaration proclaimed a need for urgent action by governments, health workers, development workers, and the entire world community to protect and promote the health of all people. It was a historic international declaration underlining the importance of primary healthcare. The primary healthcare approach has since then been accepted by most UN-member countries as the key to achieving the goal of "health for all." The document faced one primary problem, which posed an enormous obstacle to it achieving its objectives. Although theoretically sound, it was born during the Cold War in a communist country. The US did attend the convention, but the Alma Ata Declaration was initially viewed with great skepticism by the US. The fifth article, and to some extent all ten articles, was broadly misinterpreted in the west. The Declaration contains ten non-binding articles for member states, but article five was the biggest challenge. It reads as follows: Governments have a responsibility for the health of their people which can be fulfilled only by the provision of adequate health and social measures. A main social target of governments, international organizations and the whole world community in the coming decades should be the attainment by all peoples of the world by the year 2000 of a level of health that will permit them to lead a socially and economically productive life. Primary health care is the key to attaining this target as part of development in the spirit of social justice.

All governments and their respective agencies now see the document for what it is: a call to action to support (financially and technically) all peoples of the world in their struggle to achieve an improved state of health. Other articles define more clearly the theme of the entire document. This document is relevant for all who engage in global health activities because it brought focused attention on the issue of healthcare equity.

The World Development Goals

The Alma Ata was an important starting point, because it was a launching point for governments to begin working on improving the health of their populations. It brought attention to the need for strategic models of disease prevention and health care delivery for the poor. For global health volunteers, it is important to look at models of improving health, and healthcare access globally. What are the models that support global efforts to improve the health and wellbeing of people in resource-poor countries? By asking this question, we will head toward best practices in global health. It does not matter if our work is a remote bush hospital in Africa for years, or a short-term medical team outreach—integrating our work with global efforts in health is foundational for finding our way to best evidence-based practice. As we go through the rest of this book, we will discuss some ideas on how we can accomplish the aim of aligning our efforts with the big picture global health goals. There are ways even short-term global health volunteers can put concentrated effort into conforming their work to combat world health challenges. As we look at strategies on how to conform our work to fit the global community's goals for development, I think it's important to look at the goals themselves and how they came into existence. It is the goals set by the global community that gave birth to the clinical guidelines we will discuss here and in the following chapters. It is these guidelines, protocols and programs that have driven significant improvement in global health over the last 30 years.

In 2015, the global community began work on 17 specific goals known as the Sustainable Development Goals. This effort began decades ago as the Millennium Development Goals. So, before we talk about how we direct our respective efforts toward achieving the Sustainable Development Goals, we should examine the first set of development goals. Because most of the global health strategies we will discuss were created under the Millennium Development Goals.

Where did this idea of establishing international goals for development come from?

In the years following the Alma Ata, many United Nations member states began an effort to inspire change around some of the biggest challenges facing their countries. The Alma-Ata cast an immense vision to change the world for the better. For the first time, people saw that through focused, collaborative effort among nations, many of the major problems facing the world's population could be addressed.

By the 1990's, this became a movement among all 191 member states of the United Nations. The movement placed collaborative effort on the problems of extreme poverty, hunger, lack of education and illiteracy, diseases such as HIV/AIDs and malaria, environmental issues, and gender discrimination. At the UN Headquarters in New York in September 2000, the United Nations Millennium Declaration was officially signed, launching the Millennium Development Goals. It should be noted that tracking improvement in these areas began back in 1990, and earlier in some countries, even though the official declaration was not signed until 2000.

These Goals were: 1) eradicate extreme poverty and hunger, 2) the achievement of primary education of all citizens, 3) promotion of gender equality and empowering of women, 4) reduction of the global child mortality rate, 5) improve maternal health reducing maternal mortality, 6) combat diseases such as HIV/AIDS and other infectious diseases, 7) sustainability of the environment and providing safe drinking water, and 8) development of partnerships between countries to aid poor countries in development.

Were the Millennium Development Goals Reached?

Did the global community accomplish the goals it set out to achieve for beginning the new millennium? The Millennium Development Goals (MDGs) were created with the hope of achieving them by the year 2015. Under the MDGs, there were specific targets and specific indicators by which they could measure if the goals were met and to what extent. The UN did several independent evaluations and summary reports to assess if the goals were achieved and to what extent. Galatsidas and Sheehy (2015) also did an analysis and summary of the data to assess if the MDGs were met and to what extent. Below, I summarize what these evaluations discovered. To keep on topic, I am including only the MDG's 4, 5, and 6, which were specifically related to health.

MDG 4 - Reduce Child Mortality

The fourth millennium development goal to reduce under-5 mortality by two-thirds fell short, but still achieved a significant level of success. This multinational collaborative effort reduced child deaths by more than half between 1990 and 2015. More precisely, the global under-5 mortality rate decreased by 53% (50-55%). It missed the desired outcome of MDG 4, but the reductions were still a vast improvement (UNICEF, 2019). According to You, et al. (2015), two areas—the east Asia-Pacific region and Latin America/Caribbean—both achieved the MDG 4 target by 2015. Sixty-two countries achieved the two-thirds reduction in child mortality outlined in MDG 4 (UNICEF, 2019).

Progress in reducing child mortality accelerated significantly between 2000 and 2015 after the official signing of the millennium development declaration. Globally, 1 in 26 children died before reaching age five in 2018. Compared to 1 in 11 in 1990, this is genuine progress (UNICEF, 2019). Child mortality (under-5 mortality) dropped from 91 deaths per 1000 live births in 1990 to 43 per 1,000 live births in 2015. This took the annual number of under-5 deaths around the world from 12.7 million to 5.9 million.

The responsiveness of child mortality to relatively low-cost community level interventions accounts for much of the success. These interventions and strategies were developed by the WHO and UNICEF and were promoted widely. They include international strategic initiatives such as IMCI (Integrated Management of Childhood Illness), IMCM (Integrated Management of Childhood Malnutrition), and the 10-step process for inpatient care of children with malnutrition. The first two are larger country-wide strategic health programming models. However, they contain clearly delineated clinical guidelines to accomplish specific aims. These aims include: improve the skills of health workers, improve health systems, and educate the community on identifying and managing sick children. There is an important point that global health volunteers from wealthy countries need to recognize when serving in a resource poor context. Children in poor communities rarely present with one problem.

Rather, they present with multiple complex clinical problems that require integrated assessment and treatments. Integrated Management of Childhood Illness (IMCI) was created to assure all intertwined medical problems were identified and managed. More on this later.

MDG 5 - Improve Maternal Health

The fifth MGD was closely related to the MDG 4, which was a two-thirds reduction in maternal mortality by 2015. According to Bryce, Black, and Victora (2013), achieving any level of success in either the 4th or 5th millennium development goals was directly tied to improving access to health care for women. There must be strategies to help women overcome the many barriers that keep them from seeking care. Barriers preventing access to care are plentiful in low- and middle-income countries. They can be related to conditions such as economic, geographic, transportation, conflict, and gender inequity, just to name a few.

Since 1990, maternal mortality has decreased by approximately 45% globally. This is far short of the goal, but still significant progress (United Nations , 2015). The enormous challenge with addressing maternal mortality is not just about eliminating barriers to healthcare services. To adequately address the problem of maternal mortality, the health system that is accessed needs to be functional and safe with surgical services, adequate post-operative care, and blood transfusion services, etc. Such services are often not available in poor communities, making this problem much harder to address than child mortality. Most of the reduction in maternal mortality also occurred since the Millennium Development Declaration in 2000 (United Nations , 2015).

Child mortality has proven responsive to low-cost community-level health interventions. Meaning, the improvements in child mortality were not as depended on advanced health care and surgical services as improvements in maternal mortality rates. Much work still needs to be done to improve maternal health services globally, but there have been some effective strategic initiatives that have contributed to the success in maternal health — the most important of which is known as Integrated Management of Pregnancy and Childbirth (IMPAC). Like IMCI, IMPAC has components that address improvements in maternal health at the healthcare system level and at the community level. It deals with multiple integrated crucial factors in the care of pregnant patients. The strategy works by addressing aspects of care and improving access to skilled care before, during, and after pregnancy and childbirth. It focuses on health systems, health workers, as well as health promotion (World Health Organization, 2020).

The health system level

At the healthcare systems level, IMPAC focuses on improving both access to care and the quality of that care, including the quality of essential services and emergency care (World Health Organization, 2020). Achieving these aims involves working at the national health policy level as well as district level to improve the management of healthcare delivery, and infrastructure. There is significant focus on system supply chains, service delivery, healthcare financing. It also includes the assessment of local needs, in addition to monitoring and evaluation of health system performance (World Health Organization, 2020).

Building Health worker capacity

Also, like IMCI and IMCM, IMPAC works to improve healthcare provider competencies. There is an extensive but easy-to-follow set of obstetrical clinical guidelines for before, during, and after birth. It is also designed in such a way that these clinical guidelines integrate other strategic clinical protocols. It integrates clinical algorithms from programs such as the prevention of HIV mother-to-child transmission (PMTCT) or malaria treatment protocols (World Health Organization, 2020).

Community health level

As mentioned prior, barriers preventing pregnant women from accessing health services in low- and middle-income countries are numerous. Any program that addresses maternal mortality must focus on eliminating these barriers (World Health Organization, 2020). IMPAC places a significant focus on managing barriers to care for young women in poor communities such as healthcare costs and transportation. Community health workers, health promotors, and trained birth attendants also play a very important role at the community level in the strategic implementation of IMPAC (World Health Organization, 2020).

What has resulted from such initiatives?

In southern Asia, the maternal mortality decreased by 64% between 1990 and 2013 (United Nations , 2015). In Africa, maternal mortality fell by 49% (United Nations , 2015). In 2015, approximately 71% of births were assisted by trained health care workers globally (United Nations , 2015). This was nearly a 60% increase since 1990. In northern Africa, the proportion of pregnant women who received at least four antenatal visits grew significantly from 50% to 89% by 2015 (United Nations , 2015). Contraceptive usage among married women aged 15 to 49 also increased from approximately 55% in 1990 to about 64% in 2015 (United Nations , 2015). The global goal to reduce maternal mortality by two-thirds was not achieved. However, significant reductions in annual maternal deaths were made.

MDG 6 - Combat HIV/AIDS, malaria, and other diseases.

The sixth Millennium Development Goal focused on HIV/AIDS because, at the time, their spread had become one of the largest public health challenges the modern world had ever encountered. However, it included some focus on many other diseases that plague poor communities around the world like malaria and tuberculosis, which are large-scale contributors to morbidity and mortality across population groups of all ages. MDG 6 aimed to halt and reverse the spread of HIV—that was an ambitious goal that fell short. On the other hand, there was rather incredible progress in slowing the spread of HIV. New cases of HIV were reduced up to 40% between the years 2000 and 2013 (United Nations , 2015). In the beginning, 3.5 million cases were positive, a number that fell to 2.1 million by 2015 (United Nations , 2015). The accessibility to antiretroviral therapy (ART) for people living with HIV or AIDS increased significantly. Global coverage of ART reached 46% by the end of 2015 (UNAIDS, 2016).

The biggest improvement was in the world's highest prevalence region, Sub-Saharan Africa. Coverage increased in this region from 24% to 54% in just five years between 2010 and 2015, increasing the reach of ART by approximately 10.3 million people in the region (UNAIDS, 2016). Botswana, Eritrea, Kenya, Malawi, Mozambique, Rwanda, South Africa, Swaziland, Uganda, Tanzania, Zambia, and Zimbabwe all increased treatment coverage by over 25% between 2010 and 2015 (UNAIDS, 2016). The incidence rate of malaria around the world also reduced by 37%. Tuberculosis-associated mortality decreased from 45% to 41% within the years of 2000 to 2013 (United Nations , 2015).

Sustainable Development Goals

The 17 Sustainable Development Goals (SDGs) are perhaps loftier, but each has specific targets to be achieved by 2030. There is only one that is specifically related to improving health: SDG #3 - Ensure healthy lives and promote well-being for all at all ages. All the SDGs are closely related, so seeking improvements in one will drive improvements in others. The 17 Sustainable Development Goals are as follows.

- Goal 1: End poverty in all its forms everywhere

- Goal 2: End hunger, achieve food security and improved nutrition, and promote sustainable agriculture

- Goal 3: Ensure healthy lives and promote well-being for all at all ages

- Goal 4: Ensure inclusive and quality education for all and promote lifelong learning

- Goal 5: Achieve gender equality and empower all women and girls

- Goal 6: Ensure availability and sustainable management of water and sanitation for all

- Goal: 7 Ensure access to affordable, reliable, sustainable, and modern energy for all

- Goal 8: Promote sustained, inclusive and sustainable economic growth; full and productive employment; and decent work for all

- Goal 9: Build resilient infrastructure, promote inclusive and sustainable industrialization, and foster innovation

- Goal 10: Reduce inequality within and among countries

- Goal 11: Make cities and human settlements inclusive, safe, resilient, and sustainable

- Goal 12: Ensure sustainable consumption and production patterns

- Goal 13: Take urgent action to combat climate change and its impacts

- Goal 14: Conserve and sustainably use the oceans, seas, and marine resources for sustainable development

- Goal 15: Protect, restore, and promote sustainable use of terrestrial ecosystems; sustainably manage forests; combat deforestation; combat desertification; and halt and reverse land degradation and halt biodiversity loss

- Goal 16: Promote peaceful and inclusive societies for sustainable development, provide access to justice for all and build effective, accountable, and inclusive institutions at all levels

- Goal 17: Strengthen the means of implementation and revitalize the global partnership for sustainable development

At first look, most of these goals are lofty and represent almost utopian ideals that are impossible for a volunteer or organization to connect to in any meaningful way. The specific targets within each make it easier to see how these elephant-size goals can be achieved one bite at a time. We will focus in on SDG #3 for the purpose of this book. However, you can access a full list of SDGs and their targets at https:// sustainabledevelopment.un.org/

Goal 3: Ensure healthy lives and promote well-being for all at all ages
Goal 3 Targets

- 3.1 By 2030, reduce the global maternal mortality ratio to less than 70 per 100,000 live births.

- 3.2 By 2030, end preventable deaths of newborns and children under 5 years of age, with all countries aiming to reduce neonatal mortality to at least as low as 12 per 1,000 live births and under-5 mortality to at least as low as 25 per 1,000 live births.

- 3.3 By 2030, end the epidemics of AIDS, tuberculosis, malaria and neglected tropical diseases and combat hepatitis, water-borne diseases, and other communicable diseases.

- 3.4 By 2030, reduce by one third premature mortality from non-communicable diseases through prevention and treatment and promote mental health and well-being.

- 3.5 Strengthen the prevention and treatment of substance abuse, including narcotic drug abuse and harmful use of alcohol.

- 3.6 By 2030, halve the number of global deaths and injuries from road traffic accidents.

- 3.7 By 2030, ensure universal access to sexual and reproductive health-care services, including family planning, information, and education, and the integration of reproductive health into national strategies and programs.

- 3.8 Achieve universal health coverage, including financial risk protection; access to quality essential health-care services; and access to safe, effective, quality, and affordable essential medicines and vaccines for all.

- 3.9 By 2030, substantially reduce the number of deaths and illnesses from hazardous chemicals and air, water, and soil pollution and contamination.

- 3.a Strengthen the implementation of the World Health Organization Framework Convention on Tobacco Control in all countries, as appropriate

- 3.b Support the research and development of vaccines and medicines for the communicable and non-communicable diseases that primarily affect developing countries; provide access to affordable essential medicines and vaccines, in accordance with the Doha Declaration on the TRIPS Agreement and Public Health, which affirms the right of developing countries to use to the full the provisions in the Agreement on Trade-Related Aspects of Intellectual Property Rights regarding flexibilities to protect public health; and, in particular, provide access to medicines for all

- 3.c Substantially increase health financing and the recruitment, development, training, and retention of the health workforce in developing countries, especially in least developed countries and small island developing states

- 3. d Strengthen the capacity of all countries, in particular developing countries, for early warning, risk reduction, and management of national and global health risks

In the chapters to follow, we will look at some of the clinical strategies the WHO has created to address these immense challenges. They remain the only evidence-based best practices for global health initiatives.

References

Bryce, J., Black, R.E. & Victora, C.G. (2013) *Millennium Development Goals 4 and 5: progress and challenges*. BMC Med 11, 225. https://doi.org/10.1186/1741-7015-11-225

Galatsidas, A., and Sheehy, F. (2015, July 6). *What have the millennium development goals achieved?* The Guardian: https://www.theguardian.com/global-development/datablog/2015/jul/06/what-millennium-development-goals-achieved-mdgs

Lomazzi, M., Borisch, B., & Laaser, U. (2014). *The Millennium Development Goals: experiences, achievements and what's next*. Global Health Action, 7:1, DOI: 10.3402/gha.v7.23695

UN. (2015). *The Millennium Development Goals Report*. United Nations.org: https://www.un.org/millenniumgoals/2015_MDG_Report/pdf/MDG%202015%20PR%20Key%20Facts%20Global.pdf

UNICEF. (2019, September). *Under-five mortality* . Retrieved from data.unicef.org: https://data.unicef.org/topic/child-survival/under-five-mortality/

WHO (n.d.). *Millennium Development Goals (MDGs)*. World Health Organization: https://www.who.int/topics/millennium_development_goals/about/en/

You Dr., D., Hug MA, L., Ejdemyr MA, Pr, S., Idele PhD, , P., Hogan PhD, D., Mather, C., . . . Alkema PhD, L. (2015). Global, regional, and national levels and trends in under-5 mortality between 1990 and 2015, with scenario-based projections to 2030: a systematic analysis by the UN Inter-agency Group for Child Mortality Estimation. *The Lancet, 386*, 2275-2286.

Emas, R. (2015, January). The Concept of Sustainable Development: Definition and Defining Principles. United Nations' 2015 Global Sustainable Development Report. DOI: 10.13140/RG.2.2.34980.22404

Kumar, S., et al. (2016). Millennium Development Goals (MDGs) to Sustainable Development Goals (SDGs): Addressing Unfinished Agenda and Strengthening Sustainable Development and Partnership. Indian Journal of Community Medicine. 41(1): 1–4. DOI: 10.4103/0970-0218.170955

UN. (n.d.). Transforming Our World: The 2030 Agenda for Sustainable Development. United Nations: https://sustainabledevelopment.un.org/content/documents/21252030%20Agenda%20for%20Sustainable%20Development%20web.pdf

Chapter 7
Clinical Best Practice Models for Resource-poor Communities

3.3 Use clinical practice guidelines for community-based health-care initiatives

Best Practice –

a procedure that has been shown by research and experience to produce optimal results and that is established or proposed as a standard suitable for widespread adoption.

Best Evidence Based Practice for Community Healthcare

In the previous chapter, we discussed an overview of some of the WHO strategic health programs and guidelines that have made a significant impact on global health over the last 30 years. Many of these strategies have proven very successful, but Integrated Management of Childhood Illness (IMCI), is one that stands out above the others. All volunteers taking part in the care of children in low- and middle-income countries should have a basic understanding of these standards, meaning they need to be familiar with how to use the chart booklet and patient record form.

What is Integrated Management of Childhood Illness IMCI?

IMCI includes protocols on assessment, treatment, and parental counseling. IMCI also includes guidelines for treating children at the rural health outpost level and deciding what cases need referral for hospital admission. Local providers often look at medical and nursing professionals volunteering for global health initiatives as a resource of new information. Using an IMCI Chart Booklet and recording form provides volunteers an opportunity to affect the preventable causes of childhood mortality in communities. Volunteer practitioners using these protocols can also reinforce their use by local providers. Most providers trained in low- and middle-income countries have learned these guidelines, but full implementation is sometimes lagging. IMCI improves both the safety and quality of healthcare provided (Tavrow, Rukyalekere, Maganda, Ndeezi, Sebina-Zziwa, & Knebel, 2002). It is the primary model for outpatient care for children ages 0-59 months in low- and middle-income countries. The program has its limitations, and it requires modification depending on geography, specifically in high-malaria versus low-malaria regions. However, it is a very functional template for improving safety and quality of outpatient pediatric care for health centers in resource poor communities.

IMCI focuses on the well-being of the whole child. Its primary aim is to reduce death, illness, and disability and to promote improved growth and development among children under five years of age. IMCI includes both preventive and curative elements that are implemented by families, communities, and health facilities (WHO Dept. of Child

Health and Development, 2009). IMCI is a valid and effective way medical volunteers can engage in the fight to reduce child mortality globally. The IMCI strategy includes three major components:

- Improving case management skills of healthcare staff

- Improving overall health systems

- Improving family and community health practices

(WHO Dept. of Child Health and Development, 2009)

Every day, millions of families seek healthcare for their sick children, taking them to hospitals, health centers, pharmacists, doctors, and traditional healers. Surveys reveal that many sick children are often not assessed or treated properly, and the parents and caregivers of children are often poorly advised (WHO Dept. of Child Health and Development, 2009). At first-level health facilities in low- and middle-income countries, medications and equipment are often scarce, and diagnostic capabilities such as radiology and laboratory services rarely exist. In resource-poor settings, providers must rely on history along with signs and symptoms to determine disease management strategies based on the best use of resources.

These factors make providing quality care to sick children a serious challenge. The WHO and UNICEF have addressed this challenge by developing IMCI. The IMCI handbook helps providers learn how to use the guidelines to interview caretakers, recognize clinical signs, choose treatments, and provide counseling and encourage preventive care. Many health workers in the rural clinic settings of low- and middle-income countries have limited education and training. Even individuals with limited education and training can follow this algorithmic set of protocols to assess, classify, and treat children.

The complete IMCI case management process is a three-step process: 1) Assess the child 2) Classify the child's illness 3) Treat the child's illness.

Assess every child by checking first for danger signs (or possible bacterial infection in a young infant), asking questions about common conditions, examining the child, and checking nutrition and immunization status (WHO/UNICEF, 2000). Classify a child's illnesses using a color-coded triage system. Because many children in poor communities present with more than one condition, each illness is classified according to whether they require red (urgent pre-referral treatment and referral), yellow (specific medical treatment and advice), or green (simple advice on home management). After classifying all conditions, identify specific treatments for the child. Children who require urgent referral receive treatment before transfer. If a child needs treatment at home, develop an integrate plan for the child, and give the first dose of drugs in the clinic. If a child should be immunized, give immunizations (WHO/UNICEF, 2000). It is an important distinction to say IMCI classifies a child's condition; it does not diagnose. I have seen pediatricians look at the classification of pneumonia and explain how the condition is not pneumonia. They missed the point entirely. The classification of pneumonia is a huge net meant to catch all the possible respiratory pathologies that may cause a child's death. Then treat or refer them appropriately to manage all the potential causes of the child's respiratory condition. It's a shotgun approach taught to less qualified workers. Of course, physicians and practitioners will also separate and diagnose each of the child's problem after this initial triage process. The classification is a starting point that will allow coverage of the biggest potential threats. Medical professionals sometimes find the assessment/triage information remedial, but it is important to learn in order to gain an understanding of this integrated approach designed by WHO/

UNICEF. It is also important to ensure all children are assessed and managed in a way that covers all the potential life-threatening conditions. This prevents less qualified providers from getting overly focused on one problem and missing critically ill or potentially critically ill children. Use of the IMCI medical record forms and flip chart quick reference are the only way to meet these standards. IMCI is the minimum standard of care for care of children in poor communities.

On the WHO website you will find the IMCI Chart Booklet and other IMCI resources. I have also posted them on the Christian Health Service Corps website in the Clinical Resources section. There are also links to the IMCI assessment and case management videos that give a basic overview of IMCI used in an African context https://www.health-servicecorps.org/what_is_imci/ .

Is IMCI Effective?

The effectiveness of IMCI training to accomplish its aims is well documented. Chopra, Patel, Cloete, Sanders, and Peterson (2005) assessed the change in quality of care provided to ill children after implementing IMCI in Cape Town, South Africa. The study observed 21 nurses in as many clinics before and after the IMCI training in Cape Town health districts. Observations of healthcare provider before and after IMCI training, respectively, showed marked improvements. There was a marked improvement in assessment and recognition of danger signs in sick children (7% before versus 72% after), assessment of co-morbidity (integrated score 5.2 versus 8.2), rational prescribing (62% versus 84%), and starting treatment in the clinic (40% versus 70%) (Chopra et. al., 2005).

The effectiveness of IMCI computer-based training programs has also shown improvements in healthcare quality. Computer-based training of IMCI is available to share with our colleagues in low- and middle-income countries. Tavrow et al. (2002) studied 120 clinicians and nurses who provided child healthcare and desired IMCI training. "Stratification was done by type (clinician, registered nurse, enrolled nurse), and they were randomly assigned to either a standard or computer-based training group". The study demonstrated computer-based training (CBT) of IMCI was as effective as standard training but cost significantly less (Tavrow, et al., 2002). Both the standard curriculum and the computer-based training had an equivalent effect on trainees (Tavrow, et al., 2002). The influence on clinical practice and knowledge retention after three to four months was also equivalent. The CBT course was shorter, cost less, and did not require the use of as many facilitators. Luis, Robert, Mwansa, and Cesa (2008) studied IMCI implementation by health providers of multiple levels of training and found similar improvements in quality in all categories. This included IMCI-trained community health workers with minimal formal education. Their recommendations were that strategies for scaling up IMCI might include providing IMCI training to health workers with much shorter training durations.

Other evidence-based quality improvement recommendations

The following are some other ideas that represent basic quality control measures for community-based global health initiatives.

Triage

In volunteer coordinated community-based healthcare projects, triage is one of the most challenging areas. Mostly because this is where the IMCI process takes place. This usually requires having a separate IMCI area for children 0- 59 months. Use of IMCI also provides insights into the community's overall health. It gives us a compilation of individual health data can provide an exceptional snapshot of a community's disease and malnutrition prevalence. This data can then aid local health providers in designing, monitoring, and implementing community health programs. Here are some basic triage steps to include in any community healthcare initiative in a low- or middle-income country.

- We should use the IMCI assessment forms and chart booklet to guide care for pediatric patients up to 60 months of age.

- Because of reduced caloric intake and frequent parasitic infections, many children have a compromised nutritional status. Weigh, measure, graph, and classify all children under five according to IMCI guidelines and or use MUAC band on children 1 to 5 years (more on this later).

- In most communities, children 12 months and older should receive parasite medication and Vitamin Supplements according to ICMI dosing guidelines.

- Strong educational interventions are also an essential component of any community-based global health initiative to reduce preventable childhood mortality. We should teach each parent at least two of the WHO/UNICEF IMCI "danger signs" prior to leaving the clinic. Refer to the IMCI Handbook, Chart Booklet, and assessment form for what we consider a "danger sign" but here they are in short.

Danger Signs

- The child is unable to drink or breastfeed
- The child vomits all food or drink
- The child has had a seizure
- The child is lethargic or unconscious

Treating children according to IMCI guidelines

In the 2005, there were only 26 specific medications recommended by the WHO in the Integrated Management of Childhood Illness (IMCI) guidelines for community clinics in low- and middle-income countries. In the 2014 edition, that was expanded to include Antiretroviral treatment medications for children with HIV. They include the following, some of which are unfamiliar to physicians from wealthy countries or are antiquated or too dangerous to use considering much safer alternative medication choices. However, they remain the gold standard for practice in low- and middle-income countries. Drugs like chloramphenicol were abandoned decades ago in most wealthy countries, but their effectiveness and very low cost keep them in use in resource-poor communities. We will also discuss the use of a few medications (specifically, the micronutrient therapies such as iron, Vitamin A, and zinc) that need to be prescribed for children in developing countries in the following section.

WHO Child Health Formulary

1	Artemether/Lumefantrine
2	Amodiaquine Tabs (200mg)
3	Quinine (inj.) (vials) (600mg/2ml)
4	Amoxicillin Tabs (250mg)/syrup 250mg or 125/5ml
5	Chloramphenicol (inj) 1-g vials
6	Chloramphenicol syrup (600ml bottles) 125mg/5ml
7	Gentamicin vials (80mg/2ml)
8	Crystalline penicillin 100,000-unit vials
9	ORS 500-ml sachet
10	Hartmann's solution 500-ml bottles
11	Nalidixic acid (250-mg tabs)
12	Metronidazole (200-mg tabs)

13	Erythromycin (250-mg tabs)
14	Mebendazole 500-mg tabs
15	Iron 200mg
16	Cotrimoxazole (80mg:400mg)
17	Folic acid tabs (5mg)
18	Paracetamol tabs (500mg)
19	Gentian violet
20	Mycostatin (20ml)
21	Diazepam – vials
22	10% glucose half-liter bottle
23	Salbutamol (tabs) 2mg
24	Salbutamol inhaler
25	Salbutamol nebulization solution (50-ml bottle)
26	Vitamin A (soft gelatinous capsules) 100,000 and 200,000 units

(WHO/UNICEF, 2014)

Childhood Disease Prevention Strategies

According to the IMCI Chart Booklet there are five general prevention interventions for community care of children in low- and middle-income countries.

1. Immunizations

2. Parasite prophylaxis

3. Vitamin A supplementation

4. Zinc supplementation

5. Iron supplementation

(WHO/UNICEF, 2014)

This text is meant only as an overview of information, it is not a comprehensive study of treatment modalities. See specific treatment and dosing recommendations in the IMCI Chart Booklet. Note, one may be able to use it in PDF form on a tablet or computer, however it is best to print it in color and bind it. The patient recording form is in the back pages of the booklet.

You can download the IMCI Chart Booklet, on the WHO website, or from the Christian Health Service Corps website at www.healthservicecorps.org .

Immunizations

According to the WHO vaccine-preventable illnesses remain responsible for the death of approximately 1.5 million children each year (World Health Organization , 2019). This is a significant portion of the more than 5 million children who die under the age of 5 each year. However, childhood immunizations also prevent between 2 and 3 million deaths of children each year. Mostly through immunization against diphtheria, tetanus, whooping cough, and measles (World Health Organization , 2019). We are not discussing vaccine prevention of SARS-CoV-2 here. I do not include it in these numbers since we are looking specifically at childhood vaccine-preventable illnesses. At the time of this writing, in September 2021, COVID vaccinations are only available for ages 12 and older. However, since the WHO declared SARS-CoV-2 a global pandemic in March 2020, to now September 2021, we are approaching 5 million deaths globally. Since COVID vaccines rolled out in early 2021, approximately 2.3 billion people have received a full dose of the vaccine (World Health Organization, 2021). However, the impact of the SARS-CoV-2 pandemic, and its worldwide vaccination campaign, have not been without cost to childhood vaccination initiatives. UNICEF now estimates 23 million children missed out on basic vaccines through routine immunization services in 2020,

3.7 million more than in 2019. Of the approximately 17 million of the children who missed basic vaccines, most live in under-served remote places, in communities affected by conflict, or in urban slums that lack access to basic health services (World Health Organization, 2020).

Global health volunteer initiatives working in low- and middle-income countries need access to vaccinations to comply with international standards of pediatric care. This is a minimum standard of care set forth by WHO, and vaccines are available in most countries at no cost. The best way for this standard to be met is for volunteers to work under the direction of local health programs which can easily access immunizations. Volunteer groups from wealthy countries may assist local health systems reaching more remote populations. Including childhood immunizations in global health initiatives is a minimum standard that is likely only achievable in partnership with local health systems and programs. We will talk about the need for health system partnerships in more details in later chapters.

Parasite prophylaxis

Remember, many children in low- and middle-income countries receive only 50% to 75% of the daily required caloric intake for growing children, sometimes less. Parasites further compromise the nutritional status of children. The WHO standard for parasite prophylaxis is to give all children one year or older mebendazole if they have not had a dose in the previous six months (WHO/UNICEF, 2014). Give 500mg mebendazole as a single dose in clinic if 1) hookworm/ whipworm is a problem in the area in which you will work, 2) the child is one year of age or older, or 3) the child has not had a dose in the previous six months (WHO/UNICEF, 2014).

Vitamin A treatment

In malnourished, micronutrient-deficient children, Vitamin A supplementation can reduce mortality by up to 23% (Vesel, et al., 2009). Vitamin A is important in interrupting the cycle of malnutrition that makes even moderately malnourished children susceptible to death in the event of a serious illness. The vicious cycle of malnutrition and how it claims the lives of even moderately malnourished children is illustrated below. It is an important topic to consider before seeing pediatric patients in low- and middle-income countries. Malnutrition underlies more than 50% of the deaths of children under age five in low- and middle-income countries. Diarrhea, acute respiratory illness, malaria, and vaccine-preventable diseases are the primary killers of children under five, but malnutrition is often the underlying factor that precipitates the child's death.

Children in poor communities of low- and middle-income countries receive Vitamin A in much higher doses than practitioners trained in developed countries are familiar with prescribing. Active collaboration with local health authorities and record-keeping is a fundamental requirement. We will speak more about this needed collaboration in a later chapter.

- Give the first dose of Vitamin A any time after six months of age to ALL CHILDREN; thereafter, give Vitamin A every six months to ALL CHILDREN.

- Give an extra dose of Vitamin A (the same dose as for supplementation) as part of treatment if the child has measles or PERSISTENT DIARRHEA.

- If the child has had a dose of Vitamin A within the past month, DO NOT GIVE VITAMIN A.

- Always record the dose of Vitamin A given on the child's chart (i.e., AGE, VITAMIN A DOSE).

- Standard dosage for Vitamin A: Six months up to twelve months – 100,000 IU; one year and older – 200,000 IU

(WHO/UNICEF, 2014)

Zinc Supplementation

Zinc supplementation has been shown to reduce diarrhea incidence by 18% and pneumonia incidence by 41% (Vesel et al., 2009). All children age two months up to five years presenting with diarrhea should receive Zinc daily for 14 days. Refer to the IMCI Chart Booklet for exact dosages. Zinc for child health usually comes in 20-mg tabs. Children over 1 year can receive a whole tab daily for 14 days. Infant age two months up to six months receive half a tablet daily. These pills can be ground and dissolved in liquid. Show the mother how to give zinc supplements; have her verbalize and (ideally) demonstrate how to mix and give the first dose.

o Infants – dissolve tablet in a small amount of expressed breast milk, ORS (oral rehydration salts), or clean water in a cup.

o Older children – tablets can be chewed or dissolved in a small amount of clean water in a cup. However, there have been instances of children choking on albendazole and zinc tablets, so exercise caution.

(WHO/UNICEF, 2014)

Childhood Anemia

In low- and middle-income countries, childhood anemia is a manifestation of micronutrient malnutrition and is exacerbated by recurrent bouts of malaria. All children who exhibit signs of anemia should receive Iron supplementation according to IMCI child health standards. Health Books International has hemoglobin color strips to use with finger-stick blood tests available at low cost. When strips are not available, assessment of Palmar Pallor is the standard of practice promoted by WHO. It has proven superior to assessments of conjunctival or mucosal membrane evaluation for pallor. There are pictures of this type of assessment in the back appendices of the IMCI Chart Booklet (WHO/UNICEF, 2014).

Iron Supplementation

Iron supplementation has been shown to improve child development in children over age two and can have a significant effect on micronutrient-deficient children (Vesel, et al., 2009).

- Iron is also given daily for 14 days in the presence of childhood anemia. In low- and middle- income countries it is commonly available in both liquid Iron syrup (Furrous Furamate) and tablets (Ferrous Sulfate) (WHO/UNICEF, 2014).

- Refer to the IMCI Chart Booklet for weight based dosing of each form.

- In many high malaria risk areas, the oral antimalarial co-artemether is also given in the presence of anemia. Refer to the specific regional IMCI guidelines for where you will practice to determine if this applies. The co-artemether should be taken with food, but there is also a suppository form available in most malaria endemic areas (WHO/UNICEF, 2014).

Assessing for High-risk Pregnancy

We should screen every pregnant mother for signs of high-risk pregnancy including gestational diabetes, pre-eclampsia, or other issues that would deem them high-risk. These patients need to be referred to a functional obstetrical facility for ongoing prenatal care and delivery. We can achieve this aim by performing the normal prenatal care visit examination, and this should include an ultrasound if possible.

There are many portable ultrasound options now available. Sonosite makes laptop size ultrasound that does acceptable obstetrical imaging. It is available for global health initiatives for approximately 25% of the retail price through their Sound Caring program. There are two handheld point of care ultrasounds that connect to a laptop or cell phone at the time of this writing. These are the Butterfy Ultrasound, and the GE Vscan, but I believe we can expect other manufacturers to enter this market in the future. These are probably not the best option for obstetrical ultrasound, but some find them usable in this context. They are one of the few examples where something may be better than nothing.

Assessing for Malnutrition

Malnutrition underlies more than 50% of child deaths in low-and middle- income countries. This makes assessment of all children for malnutrition essential. The malnutrition and disease cycle demonstrates how even children who are moderately malnourished, can progress to decompensation and death in a relatively short amount of time.

Malnutrition and Disease Cycle

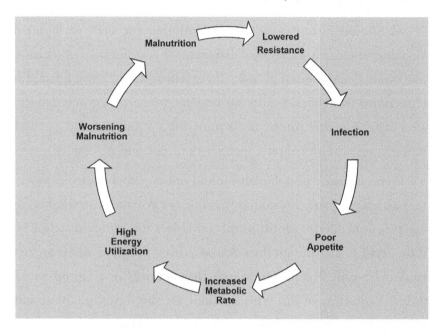

Malnutrition Assessment Standards

The WHO and UNICEF (2009) document entitled "Child growth standards and the identification of severe acute malnutrition in infants and children" defines how all children under the age of five should be assessed at each encounter with a healthcare professional. Middle upper-arm circumference (MUAC) predicts mortality better than any other measure. In children between the ages of 18 months and 60 months, MUAC and weight-for-height are roughly equivalent in their diagnostic and prognostic values. When assessing children for malnutrition using weight-for-height, the WHO and UNICEF recommend the use of a cut-off of below -3 standard deviations (SD) from the mean to classify a child with severe acute malnutrition (SAM). The commonly used cut-off is the same for both the 2006 WHO child growth standards and the earlier National Center for Health Statistics (NCHS reference). According to the WHO and UNICEF (2009), the reasons for the choice of this cut-off are: (a) children below this cut-off have a highly elevated risk of death compared to those who are above it; (b) these children have a higher weight gain when receiving a therapeutic diet compared to other diets, which results in faster recovery; (c) in a well-nourished population, there are virtually no children below -3 SD (<1%); and (d) there are no known risks or negative effects associated with the therapeutic feeding of these children applying recommended protocols and appropriate therapeutic foods (WHO and UNICEF, 2009).

Middle Upper Arm Circumference MUAC

Color-coded middle-upper-arm-circumference (MUAC) bands that measure to the millimeter make classifying malnourished children according to WHO standards easier with less potential for error. UNICEF has them available to order and a simple search for MUAC bands will usually reveal places from which they can be purchased. Christian Health Service Corps has created MUAC bands and make them available to staff, health program partners and volunteers.

- We usually assess height, weight and head circumference for all children younger than 1 year of age. Children 12 months to 59 months can be assessed using a MUAC band. It can be used in children as early as six months with arm length greater than 65 cm.

- Children should also be examined for signs of visible wasting and assessed for signs of pitting edema in the distal extremities and forehead.

- Children exhibiting signs of visible wasting, pitting edema, or MUAC measurement less than 13.5 cm need admission to a therapeutic re-feeding program. Usually inpatient, but this depend on availability of services in the region. Community based therapeutic refeeding may initially be the only option without transferring children a significant distance.

- Xerophthalmia screening and treatment, if necessary, should be done for all children in regions where there is a high malnutrition prevalence.

The website Mother and Child Nutrition - see http://motherchild-nutrition.org/ is an exceptional resource for learning strategies for community-based nutritional assessment.

Remember malnutrition may look very different depending on the age of the child, available food sources, and if the child is still breast-feeding. In Marasmus (dry malnutrition), the child exhibits severe visible wasting. In Kwashiorkor's (wet malnutrition), where edema is present, it is sometimes harder to spot because the child may weigh normally, and look normal at first glance. However, assessing for pitting edema of the forehead and extremities will keep you from missing this pathology. Children with chronic forms of malnutrition may have stunting, severe anemia and are still at high mortality risk during severe illness.

Standards for Inpatient Care of Children with Severe Acute Malnutrition

The WHO has outlined a 10-step protocol for the care and therapeutic re-feeding of patients. Inpatient treatment of a child with severe acute malnutrition usually takes between 2 to 6 weeks.

		PHASE		
		STABILISATION		REHABILITATION
Step		Days 1-2	Days 3-7	Weeks 2-6
1. Hypoglycaemia		——→		
2. Hypothermia		——→		
3. Dehydration		——→		
4. Electrolytes		—————————————————→		
5. Infection		——————————→		
6. Micronutrients			no iron	with iron ——→
7. Cautious feeding		————————→		
8. Catch-up growth				——————————→
9. Sensory stimulation		—————————————————→		
10. Prepare for follow-up				——————————→

However, if the community support is available close to where the child lives, they may be discharged early (at step 8) to continue recovery at home. These steps are broken into two phases. The first phase is the stabilization phase, where acute medical problems are managed. The second phase is and a longer rehabilitation phase.

Below summarizes the 10 steps for inpatient care of children with severe acute malnutrition:

- Treat/ prevent hypoglycemia - Treat hypoglycemia with glucose immediately. Feeding malnourished children every 2-3 hours around the clock To prevent hypoglycemia.

- Treat/prevent hypothermia - To treat hypothermia by actively re-warming the child, and keep malnourished children warm.

- Treat/prevent dehydration - Too much fluid can kill. Rehydrate more slowly than usual. Do not give IV fluids except in shock.

- Correct electrolyte imbalance - Give extra potassium and magnesium daily. Limit sodium (salt).

- Treat/prevent infection - Give antibiotics routinely to all severely malnourished children to treat hidden infections and prevent death. Wash hands to prevent cross-infection.

- Correct micronutrient deficiencies - Give extra vitamin A, zinc, copper, folic acid and multivitamins. Do not give iron until the child is in the rehabilitation phase.

- Start cautious feeding - Give small amounts of F75 every 3 hours day and night. F75 is a special formula designed to meet the needs of malnourished children.

- Achieve catch-up growth - For rapid weight gain, give as much F100 or ready-to-use therapeutic food (RUTF) as the child can eat, 8 times a day. F100 and RUTF are high in energy and protein.

- Provide sensory stimulation and emotional support - Provide loving care, play and stimulation to improve mental development.

- Prepare for follow-up after recovery - Teach mothers what to feed at home to help the child recover. Malnourished children need regular follow-up to prevent relapse and death.

(Ashworth, Khanum, Jackson, & Schofield, 2003)

You can download the Guidelines for the inpatient treatment of severely malnourished children directly from the WHO website, or CHSC Website resource page at www.healthservicecorps.org

References

Ashworth, A., Khanum, S., Jackson, A., & Schofield, C. (2003). *Guidelines for the inpatient treatment of severely malnourished children.* Geneva: World Health Organization .

Chopra, M., Patel, S., Cloete, K., Sanders, D., & Peterson, S. (2005). Effect of an IMCI intervention on quality of care across four districts in Cape Town, South Africa. *Archives of Disease in Childhood, 90,* 397–401.

Luis, H., Robert, S., A Mwansa, N., & Cesa, R. V. (2008). How much does quality of care vary between health workers with different levels of training? An observational multi-country study. *The Lancet, Research Library Core, 372,* 910–916.

Tavrow, P., Rukyalekere, A., Maganda, A., Ndeezi, G., Sebina-Zziwa, A., & Knebel, E. (2002). *A comparison of computer-based and standard training in the integrated management of childhood illness in Uganda.* Bethesda: USAID by the Quality Assurance Project, University Research Co.

WHO Dept. of Child Health and Development. (2009, January). Child and adolescent health topics. Retrieved from http://www.who.int/child_adolescent_health/topics/prevention_care/child/imci/en/

WHO Secretary General. (2008). *Progress report on millennium development goals.* New York: United Nations Department of Economic and Social Affairs. Retrieved from http://www.un.org/millenniumgoals/pdf/The%20Millennium%20Development%20Goals%20Report%202008.pdf

WHO and UNICEF . (2009). *Child growth standards and the identification of servere acute malnutrition in infants.* Geneva: WHO.

WHO/UNICEF. (2014). *IMCI Handbook.* Geneva: WHO Press.

World Health Organization . (2019). *Immunization Facts.* Retrieved from World Health Organization : https://www.who.int/news-room/facts-in-pictures/detail/immunization

World Health Organization . (2020). *Immunization Agenda 2030: A global strategy to leave no one behind.* Geneva: World Health Organization.

World Health Organiztion . (2021, September 15). *WHO Coronavirus (COVID-19) Dashboard.* Retrieved from World Health Organization: https://covid19.who.int/

Chapter 8
Improving Surgical Safety in Global Health

3.4. Use clinical practice guidelines for surgical initiatives

3.5. Assess Operating Room Capacity and Safety

3.4. Use clinical practice guidelines for surgical initiatives

Ensuring adherence to clinical practice guidelines, clinical pathways, and other evidence-based recommendations could not have more value than it does in short-term surgical initiatives. Few if any global health initiatives have as much to offer as surgical initiatives; however, they also represent the highest potential for adverse outcomes. The potential for tragic outcomes can be decreased significantly by simply following the WHO safe surgery protocols, checklists, and current evidence-based recommendations for surgical safety in developing countries. The WHO World Alliance for Patient Safety (2009) "Guidelines for Safe Surgery" outline the critical aspects of surgical safety in all countries. This document can be downloaded from the WHO website along with the safe surgery checklist and infra-structure requirements for safe surgery. There are 10 essential objectives for the WHO safe surgery guidelines, which are:

Objective 1: Operate on the correct patient at the correct site.

Objective 2: Use methods known to prevent harm from ad-ministration of anesthetics while protecting the patient from pain.

Objective 3: Recognize and effectively prepare for life-threat-ening loss of airway

or respiratory function.

Objective 4: Recognize and effectively prepare for risk of high blood loss.

Objective 5: Avoid inducing an allergic or adverse drug reac-tion for which the patient is known to be at significant risk.

Objective 6: Consistently use methods known to minimize the risk for surgical site infection.

Objective 7: Prevent inadvertent retention of instruments and sponges in surgical wounds.

Objective 8: Secure and accurately identify all surgical speci-mens.

Objective 9: Communicate and exchange critical information for surgical safety.

Objective 10: Hospitals and public health systems will estab-lish routine surveillance of surgical capacity, volume, and re-sults.

(WHO World Alliance for Patient Safety, 2009, p. 10)

The WHO Guidelines for Safe Surgery are designed to meet these 10 objectives and are organized in three sections. They have been developed based on clinical evidence and expert opinion and are categorized based on their ability to reduce the likelihood of serious, avoidable surgical complications or adverse events. The three categories are as follows:

1) **Highly Recommended**: a practice that should be in place for each and every surgery.

2) **Recommended**: a practice that is encouraged for each and every surgery.

3) **Suggested**: a practice that should be considered for any surgery.

(WHO World Alliance for Patient Safety, 2009, p. 7)

The following are considered **highly recommended** for peri-operative and peri-anesthesia care by the WHO.

1) Continuous presence of a vigilant, professionally trained anesthesia provider. If an emergency requires the brief, temporary absence of the primary anesthetist, judgment must be exercised in comparing the threat of an emergency to the risk of the anaesthetized patient's condition and in selecting the clinician left responsible for anesthesia during the temporary absence.

2) Supplemental oxygen should be supplied for all patients undergoing general anesthesia. Tissue oxygenation and perfusion should be monitored continuously using a pulse oximeter with a variable-pitch pulse tone loud enough to be heard throughout the operating room.

3) The adequacy of the airways and of ventilation should be monitored continuously by observation and auscultation. When-

ever mechanical ventilation is employed, a disconnect alarm should be used.

4) Circulation should be monitored continuously by auscultation or palpation of the heartbeat or by a display of the heart rate on a cardiac monitor or pulse oximeter.

5) Arterial blood pressure should be determined at least every 5 minutes and more frequently if indicated by clinical circumstances.

6) A means of measuring body temperature should be available and used at frequent intervals where clinically indicated (e.g., prolonged or complex anesthesia, children).

7) The depth of anesthesia (degree of unconsciousness) should be assessed regularly by clinical observation.

(WHO World Alliance for Patient Safety, 2009, p. 25)

The following are considered **recommended** for peri-operative and peri-anesthesia care by the WHO.

1) Inspired oxygen concentration should be monitored throughout anesthesia with an instrument fitted with a low oxygen-concentration alarm. In addition, a device to protect against the delivery of a hypoxic gas mixture and an oxygen supply-failure alarm should be used.

2) Continuous measurement and display of the expired carbon dioxide waveform and concentration (capnography) should be used to confirm the correct placement of an endotracheal tube and the adequacy of ventilation.

3) The concentrations of volatile agents should be measured continuously, as should inspiratory or expired gas volumes.

4) An electrocardiograph should be used to monitor heart rate and rhythm.

5) A cardiac defibrillator should be available.

6) Body temperature should be measured continuously in patients in whom a change is anticipated, intended, or suspected. This can be done by continuous electronic temperature measurement, if available.

7) A peripheral nerve stimulator should be used to assess the state of paralysis when neuromuscular-blocking drugs are given.

(WHO World Alliance for Patient Safety, 2009, p. 25)

Surgical Safety Checklist

The Alliance for Patient Safety estimates there are 7 million disabling surgical complications and 1 million surgical-related deaths worldwide each year. They identify three primary problems with surgical safety: (a) it is unrecognized as a public health issue, (b) there is a lack of data on surgery and outcomes (especially in developing countries), and (c) there is a failure to use existing safety know-how. In an attempt to improve surgical safety, they launched the *Safe Surgery Saves Lives* campaign. The centerpiece of this program is a checklist known as the Surgical Safety Checklist (WHO World Alliance for Patient Safety, 2009). In order to develop the WHO Surgical Safety Checklist, the authors used the aviation industry checklist framework because of the industry's more than half century of experience in developing and using checklists to improve safety. The checklist has proven to be a great success: eight hospitals from both developed and developing countries participated in a study, and the checklist was shown to improve adherence to standards of care by 65% and reduce surgical-related mortality by half (Weiser et al., 2010).

The checklist has three sections: before induction of anesthesia, before skin incision, and before the patient leaves the operating room (WHO Alliance for Patient Safety, 2008). The advantages to using the checklist include the following: (a) it can be customized to the local setting, (b) it is strongly evidence-based, (c) it has been evaluated in both developed and developing countries with similar results, (d) it promotes adherence to known best practices, and (e) it does not require significant resources to implement (WHO World Alliance for Patient Safety, 2009).

It is considered **highly recommended** for any program involving surgical care of patients to use the WHO Surgical Safety Checklist; in fact, it is best considered a minimum standard of care. The checklist shown here is for illustration and reference purposes only. It is recommended that any facility or program doing surgery go to the WHO webpage for surgical safety, download the PDF version, and make enough copies to have one for each surgical case. It is also recommended that a copy of the checklist be attached to the permanent patient record.

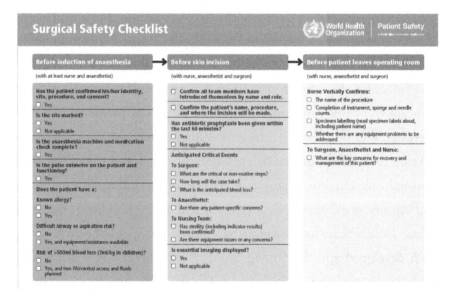

Image used for educational reference purposes (WHO, 2009). To download copies for use, see http://www.who.int/patientsafety/safesurgery/en/index.html.

Of the 234 million people who undergo surgery each year, approximately one million of these individuals die from surgical complications. The WHO estimates that expanded use of the checklist could prevent more than half of these deaths (WHO World Alliance for Patient Safety, 2009). The following is an overview of each section of the Surgical Safety Checklist. What appears here is only a brief summary of the steps to using the WHO Surgical Safety Checklist. It is recommended that readers download a copy of the WHO Surgical Safety Implementation Guide. A complete list of safe surgery tools, the checklist, an implementation manual, and other resources can be found at http://www.who.int/patientsafety/safesurgery/tools_resources/en/index.html. A video demonstration on the use of the WHO Surgical Safety Checklist can be found at http://www.safesurg.org/how-to.html.

Sign-in phase prior to the induction of anesthesia

At sign-in - The person coordinating the checklist will verbally review with the patient (when possible):

1) Their identity

2) That the procedure and site are correct and that consent for surgery has been given

3) The coordinator will visually confirm that the operative site has been marked and that a pulse oximeter is on the patient and functioning.

4) The checklist coordinator will also verbally review with the anesthesia professional the patient's risk of blood loss, airway difficulty, and allergic reaction, and whether a full anesthesia safety check has been completed.

5) Ideally, the surgeon will be present for sign-in, as the surgeon may have a clearer idea of anticipated blood loss, allergies, or other complicating patient factors.

(WHO Alliance for Patient Safety, 2008)

Before induction of anaesthesia

(with at least nurse and anaesthetist)

Has the patient confirmed his/her identity, site, procedure, and consent?
☐ Yes

Is the site marked?
☐ Yes
☐ Not applicable

Is the anaesthesia machine and medication check complete?
☐ Yes

Is the pulse oximeter on the patient and functioning?
☐ Yes

Does the patient have a:

Known allergy?
☐ No
☐ Yes

Difficult airway or aspiration risk?
☐ No
☐ Yes, and equipment/assistance available

Risk of >500ml blood loss (7ml/kg in children)?
☐ No
☐ Yes, and two IVs/central access and fluids planned

Timeout before skin incision

The timeout requires that all team members introduce themselves and state their role. The team can simply confirm that everyone in the room is known to each other if more than one case is being done by the same team.

Prior to the skin incision, the team must pause and confirm aloud that they are performing the correct operation on the correct patient, and on the correct site.

They must then review aloud with one another the critical elements of plans for the operation using the checklist questions for guidance.

It must also be confirmed that prophylactic antibiotics have been given within the previous 60 minutes and that imaging is displayed, when appropriate.

(WHO Alliance for Patient Safety, 2008)

Sign-out

Once sign-out is initiated, the nurse verbally confirms with all team members:

1. The name of the procedure recorded

2. That the instrument, needle, and sponge counts are correct and reconciled prior to closure

3. If counts are not reconciled, the team is alerted to search for missing items in, on, or around the field. X-rays are requested if counts still do not reconcile.

(WHO Alliance for Patient Safety, 2008)

Before skin incision

(with nurse, anaesthetist and surgeon)

☐ Confirm all team members have introduced themselves by name and role.

☐ Confirm the patient's name, procedure, and where the incision will be made.

Has antibiotic prophylaxis been given within the last 60 minutes?
☐ Yes
☐ Not applicable

Anticipated Critical Events

To Surgeon:
☐ What are the critical or non-routine steps?
☐ How long will the case take?
☐ What is the anticipated blood loss?

To Anaesthetist:
☐ Are there any patient-specific concerns?

To Nursing Team:
☐ Has sterility (including indicator results) been confirmed?
☐ Are there equipment issues or any concerns?

Is essential imaging displayed?
☐ Yes
☐ Not applicable

Before patient leaves operating room

(with nurse, anaesthetist and surgeon)

Nurse Verbally Confirms:
☐ The name of the procedure
☐ Completion of instrument, sponge and needle counts
☐ Specimen labelling (read specimen labels aloud, including patient name)
☐ Whether there are any equipment problems to be addressed

To Surgeon, Anaesthetist and Nurse:
☐ What are the key concerns for recovery and management of this patient?

3.5. Assess Operating Room Capacity and Safety

Schneider et al.'s (2011) "Volunteers in plastic surgery guidelines for providing surgical care of children in the less developed world" outlines 10 guidelines that closely parallel the WHO safety guidelines; however, they were developed from the perspective of surgical providers who practice in developed countries. They address considerations that providers trained in developing countries will automatically consider, such as the ramifications of operating on malnourished children and the delayed healing process. Failure of providers from developed countries to consider such issues has resulted in reported child deaths (Garbern, 2010). They also address the need for a facility site visit to ensure adequate healthcare infrastructure to perform surgery safely. Needle stick HIV chemoprophylaxis is also included in this set of guidelines, and this is considered an important consideration for global health surgical volunteers.

Infrastructure assessment is a vital aspect of setting up a safe global surgical initiative. According to the WHO World Alliance for Patient Safety (2009), medical facilities are divided into three levels, with each having defined equipment requirements. Level 1 facilities are small hospitals or health centers, and they should meet at least "highly recommended" anesthesia standards. Level 2 facilities are district or provincial facilities, and they should meet at least "highly recommended" and "recommended" anesthesia standards. Level 3 facilities are referral facilities, and they should meet at least "highly recommended," "recommended," and "suggested" anesthesia standards. The following are the equipment and infrastructure expected for the respective facility levels of care. However, it is important to note that although these are expected standards, many facilities lack even the most basic infrastructure for safe surgery. One cannot assume that just because a facility has a level designation it is anywhere close to meeting recommended safety and equipment requirements, making a site visit for patient safety infrastructure a requirement for surgical initiatives. The following lists were taken directly from the WHO Alliance for Patient Safety Guidelines for safe surgery. They have been modified here into infrastructure checklists for surgical providers and project leaders to use during their pre-project site assessment. It is recommended that global surgical programs partner with Level 2 or Level 3 facilities to achieve optimal levels of patient safety. Facility and site assessment should take place months before the planned surgical project. The WHO equipment and medication lists below should be used to assist in the final site approval. If a facility is a Level 1, but infrastructure can be supplemented with equipment and medication by the visiting group, this is acceptable. The existing infrastructure, the team's ability to improve the infrastructure, consistency of power supply, consistency of oxygen supply, and functionality of anesthesia equipment should all be taken into consideration in the final site approval. Many facilities have equipment that has not been used for some time or at all, and it is therefore important to make sure not only that the equipment is there, but also that it is functioning properly. Consequently, it is ideal that an anesthesia provider complete the surgical site assessment whenever possible. Other medications and equipment highly recommended for global health surgical initiatives that are not included in the WHO medication and infrastructure list include (a) a malignant hyperthermia treatment kit with dantrolene and (b) an HIV needle stick chemoprophylaxis for team members.

Level 1	Level 2	Level 3
Small hospital or health center (Should meet at least "highly recommended" anesthesia standards)	District or provincial hospital (Should meet at least "highly recommended" and "recommended" anesthesia standards)	Referral hospital (Should meet at least "highly recommended," "recommended," and "suggested" anesthesia standards)

Equipment	Equipment	Equipment
□ Adult and pediatric self-inflating breathing bags with masks	**The same as Level 1 plus the following complete anesthesia, resuscitation, and airway-management systems, including:**	**Same as Level 2 with these additions (per each per operating room or intensive care unit bed, except where stated):**
□ Foot-powered suction stethoscopes	□ Reliable oxygen sources	□ Anesthesia ventilator, reliable electric power source with manual override
□ Sphygmomanometers	□ Vaporizer(s)	
□ and thermometers	□ Hoses and valves	□ Infusion pumps (two per bed),
□ Pulse oximeter	□ Bellows or bag to inflate lungs	
□ Oxygen concentrator or tank oxygen and a draw-over vaporizer with hoses	□ Face masks (sizes 00–5)	□ pressure bag for intravenous infusion
	□ Work surface and storage	
□ Laryngoscopes, bougies	□ Pediatric anesthesia system	□ Electric or pneumatic suction
	□ Oxygen supply failure alarm; oxygen analyzer	□ Oxygen analyzer*
	□ Adult and pediatric resuscitator sets	□ Thermometer (temperature probe*)
	□ Pulse oximeter, spare probes, adult and pediatric capnograph	□ Electric warming blanket
		□ Electric overhead heater
	□ Defibrillator (one per operating suite or intensive care unit)	□ Infant incubator
		□ Laryngeal mask, airways sizes (three sets per operating room)
	□ Electrocardiograph monitor	
	□ Laryngoscope, Macintosh blades 1–3(4)	□ Intubating bougies, adult and child (one set per operating room)
	□ Oxygen concentrator(s) (cylinder)	□ Anesthetic agent (gas and vapor) analyzer
	□ Foot or electric suction	
	□ Intravenous pressure bag	□ Depth-of-anesthesia monitors are being increasingly recommended for cases at high risk of awareness but are not standard in many countries.
	□ Adult and pediatric resuscitator sets	
	□ Magill forceps (adult and child)	
	□ Intubation stylet or bougie	
	□ Spinal needles 25G	
	□ Nerve stimulator	
	□ Automatic non-invasive blood pressure monitor	

Disposable	Disposable	Disposable
□ Examination gloves	**Same as Level 1 with the following additions:**	**Same as Level 2 with the following additions:**
□ Intravenous infusion and drug injection equipment	□ EKG electrodes	□ Ventilator circuits
□ Suction catheters, size 16 FG	□ Intravenous equipment (minimum fluids: normal saline, Ringer lactate. and dextrose 5%)	□ Yankauer suckers
□ Airway support equipment, including airways and tracheal tubes		□ Sets for intravenous infusion pumps
□ Oral and nasal airways	□ Pediatric IV sets	□ Disposables for suction machines
	□ Suction catheters, size 16 FG	□ Disposables for capnography, oxygen analyzer, in accordance with manufacturers' specifications:
	□ Sterile gloves, sizes 6–8	
	□ Nasogastric tubes, sizes 10–16 FG	
	□ Oral airways, sizes 000–4	□ Sampling lines
	□ Tracheal tubes sizes 3–8.5 mm	□ Water traps
		□ Connectors
	□ Spinal needles sizes 22 G and 25G, Batteries size C	□ Filters and fuel cells

Equipment list formatted as a checklist for surgical global health initiatives (WHO World Alliance for Patient Safety, 2009, pp. 22-24).

Level 1	Level 2	Level 3
Small hospital or health center (Should meet at least "highly recommended" anesthesia standards)	District or provincial hospital (Should meet at least "highly recommended" and "recommended" anesthesia standards)	Referral hospital (Should meet at least "highly recommended," "recommended," and "suggested" anesthesia standards)
Medication	**Medication**	**Medication**
☐ Ketamine 50mg/ml injection ☐ Lidocaine 1% or 2% ☐ Diazepam ☐ Midazolam injection ☐ Pethidine injection ☐ Morphine ☐ Epinephrine ☐ Atropine ☐ Appropriate inhalation ☐ Anesthetic if vaporizer	**Same as Level 1, but with the following additions:** ☐ Thiopental or propofol ☐ Suxamethonium bromide ☐ Pancuronium ☐ Neostigmine ☐ Ether, halothane, or other inhalation anesthetics ☐ Lidocaine 5% heavy spinal solution, 2ml ☐ Bupivacaine 0.5% ☐ Hydralazine 20mg injection ☐ Furosemide injection ☐ Dextrose 50% injection ☐ Aminophylline injection ☐ Ephedrine ampoules ☐ Hydrocortisone	**Same as Level 2 with the following additions:** ☐ Propofol ☐ Nitrous oxide ☐ Various modern neuromuscular blocking agents ☐ Various modern inhalation anesthetics ☐ Various inotropic agents ☐ Various intravenous antiarrhythmic agents ☐ Nitroglycerine for infusion ☐ Calcium chloride 10% 10-ml injection ☐ Potassium chloride 20% 10-ml injection for infusion

List formatted as a checklist for surgical global health initiatives

(WHO World Alliance for Patient Safety, 2009, pp. 22-24).

In the next chapter, we will look at the design, monitoring, and evaluation (DME) of global health initiatives in the larger program context.

References

Garbern, S. C. (2010). Medical relief trips...what's missing? Exploring the ethical issues and the physician-patient relationship. *Einstein Journal of Biology and Medicine*, 38–40.

Weiser, T. G., Haynes, A. B., Lashoher, A., Dzeikan, G., Boorman, D. J., Berry, W. R. (2010). Perspectives in quality: Designing the WHO surgical safety checklist. *International Journal of Quality in Healthcare*, 365–70.

WHO Alliance for Patient Safety. (2008) *Implementation manual for surgical safety checklist.* Geneva: WHO Alliance for Patient Safety.

WHO World Alliance for Patient Safety. (2009). *WHO guidelines for safe surgery.* Geneva: WHO.

Chapter 9
Medical Records

Best Practice Guideline 4
Complete and thorough documentation on each patient

4.1 Document assessment, plan of care, and the care provided.

4.2 Document all relevant information relating to the patient's condition, to interventions, and to actions taken.

4.3 Document standard of care for the context.

4.4 Documentation should provide evidence that the clinician met his/her duty of care and that any errors or omissions did not compromise patient safety or identified health outcomes.

4.5 Documentation should include any communication shared with patient or family in the way of treatment, condition, or health education and counseling.

4.6 Perform quality assurance reviews of documentation.

4.7 Provide copies of patient medical records to local services or those responsible for follow-up care.

Best Practice Guideline 4

Document All Healthcare Provided

No provider or organization is exempt from documentation of their clinical practice in the provision of healthcare services. Clinical documentation is a minimum standard for all healthcare services in all countries. The World Health Organization in their document "Guidelines for medical record and clinical documentation" defines this standard. This WHO document describes three guiding principles for documentation, which are:

1) Comprehensive, complete medical records - Clinical staff have a professional obligation to maintain documentation that is clear, concise, comprehensive, and true.

2) Patient-centered and collaborative - Documentation is patient-centered, patient-focused, collaborative, and appropriate to the clinical setting.

3) Ensure and maintain patient confidentiality - Documentation systems must ensure and maintain patient confidentiality.

In this document, the WHO refers to clinical documentation as a fundamental part of clinical practice. Documentation provides a record of health services for other providers to follow. It also holds the clinician's accountable to standards of care (WHO-South East Asia Office, 2007). Dohn and Dohn's (2003) study on the healthcare quality of volunteer healthcare projects cites lack of or poor quality documentation as a significant barrier to achieving quality in global health initiatives. Without complete, accurate documentation, patient safety is not achievable according to the WHO safety framework (WHO World Alliance for Patient Safety, 2009). Documentation is used to evaluate professional practice within quality assurance programs, such as process reviews, adherence to standards, audits, credentialling, and critical incident reviews (WHO-South East Asia Office, 2007).

The purposes of the WHO clinical documentation guidelines include quality improvement, healthcare provider accountability, and fulfilling legislative requirements that exist in most countries, as well as retrospective healthcare audits and research. I took the first five of the seven subsections of this best practice guideline 4 directly from the WHO document "Guidelines for medical record and clinical documentation". Therefore, those individual rationales are not discussed separately since they reflect current known international standards for healthcare. They are standards that apply to both permanent and temporary healthcare delivery programs, regardless of global geography.

4.6. Review all patient records to assure quality of care

Review all patient records for completeness and adherence to safety standards. Volunteer medical projects must establish a system of record review either directly or through their local health system partners. This process should be noted in the patient safety policy of global health organizations. Medical record documentation tells us much about a program's commitment to quality and patient safety. Dohn and Dohn (2003), in their assessment of the quality of healthcare teams in the Dominican Republic, reported that some volunteer teams asked fewer than 15% of patients about allergies. Their records showed that 700 of the patients had no notation of when the patient last saw a physician. It was believed by most volunteers that there was little or no access to healthcare by the population being served. Yet follow-up surveys revealed 42% of the patients had seen a local physician in the three months prior to visit of the medical volunteers.

4.7. Provide copies of medical records to follow up providers

According to the WHO guidelines for clinical documentation, medical records are essential for the inter-professional communication necessary to avoid medical errors and achieve patient safety (WHO-South East Asia Office, 2007). Most medical volunteers from wealthy countries are not going to areas that are extremely remote where there are no healthcare facilities. Medical records created by volunteer providers should be integrated into the permanent patient medical record where one exists. As much as possible, write medical records in the language of the local medical community. However, many physician providers in other countries have some English skills. Documentation of care provided by international volunteers should be accessible to ensure the continuity of care for each patient.

References

Dohn, M. N., & Dohn A. L. (2003). Quality of care on short-term medical missions: Experience with a standardized medical record and related issues. *Missiology: An International Review,* 417–429.

WHO-South East Asia Office. (2007). *Guidelines for medical record and clinical documentation.* New Delhi: WHO.

WHO World Alliance for Patient Safety. (2009). *Conceptual framework for the international classification for patient safety.* Geneva: World Health Organization.

Chapter 10
Poverty, Paternalism, Ownership, and Control

"Poverty is not just a lack of money; it is not having the capability to realize one's full potential as a human being."

- Abhijit V. Banerjee

Best Practice Guideline 5
Build Capacity

The Lion Story

There was once a rural community in Africa that was having a problem with lion attacks. This had not occurred in many years, and it started again suddenly. One night, a lion came into the village and killed and carried off a man. Initially, it was assumed this was a one-time event because it had been at least 50 years since the last time this had occurred. However, a few nights later, the lion returned, killing and taking a child. Then it happened again a few nights later. This cycle went on; every few nights, the lion would come to the village and feed.

The villagers got together and decided to send a delegation by bus to the government office in the city for help. They were assured the regional game warden would be dispatched, so they returned home. But help never came, and the problem continued.

The community met again and decided to ask for help from an aid organization a few communities away. The aid program said they would help, and they held meetings about how to solve the lion problem for the village. The agency decided that they should put up battery-powered lights with motion sensors that would scare away the lion. It took a few weeks to complete, but once they were up, everyone felt this would be the answer to the lion problem. The lights worked initially, but after a short time, they did not scare the lion, and it continued feeding in the village.

The people of the village then decided to meet with another aid organization. This one also agreed to help, and after having several meetings, this agency decided they would put up sirens with the lights, which would be certain to scare the lion away. It worked for a few weeks, but the lion became less and less afraid of the sirens and resumed its pattern of stalking villagers after dark.

Frustrated and disheartened, the villagers sent another delegation, this time to a much bigger aid organization in a faraway city. They also agreed to rescue the village. This aid organization also held several meetings and decided the best thing to do to help the villagers was to build a fence around the entire village for protection. This took a few months to complete, but when it was constructed, the village had a big celebration because the lion could no longer enter the village at night. The village was peaceful for several weeks after the fence was constructed, and everyone was finally beginning to relax since the danger was controlled. One morning, the village women and children went to collect water at the river outside the village as they did every morning. The lion attacked and killed a child. This became its new pattern, waiting for the women to gather water in the morning.

The villagers had yet another meeting, and one of the community elders said that when this happened many years ago, the men of the village would hunt the lions. He suggested they speak with the one man in the community that was still alive who had hunted the lions. When they met with the very elderly man, he asked why they had not sought his advice before because he could teach the young men of the community how to hunt and kill the lion. He trained the young men for a few days, and they were then able to hunt and kill the lion within a week.

5.1. Surrender Ownership and Control to the Community

The starting point for best practice guideline - 5 Build Capacity - is to surrender ownership and control of our projects and programs to local communities. However, to understand the reason for this, it's important to outline some underlying concepts in cross-cultural work. The Lion Story helps us discover some of these concepts.

The original author of the Lion Story is unknown, but it was first told to me in a community development workshop while I was serving with Mercy Ships International. It is a story every global health organization and volunteer needs to hear. There are many lions in resource-poor communities around the world. Sometimes the lions look like maternal mortality, childhood malnutrition, HIV, TB, or malaria. The important takeaway is that the answer to the lion problem will always come from within the community. As an outsider, we can only serve and support their efforts to hunt and kill their lions. In the last chapter I talked about health education — in this chapter we will transition into the need for *Best Practice Guideline 5 - Build Capacity* which starts with surrendering ownership and control to the community. Our role in global health is to help the community realize that they have the answers to the lion problem, and they are strong enough to kill the lions.

The Lion Story exemplifies the classic pattern of paternalism exhibited by well-intentioned organizations and their volunteers still to this day. Paternalism is the attitude of a person who subordinates another as if they should be controlled in a fatherly way for their own good. Paternalism degrades self-worth because it involves treating others as children and implying that they are not qualified to decide things for themselves. Fortunately, most professional relief and development organizations have learned how to avoid paternalism. However, global health programs, universities, and charities and volunteers often fall into the paternalism trap. Even long-term medical workers can fall into this trap. I know of two hospitals started by American organizations that, after years of operation, still do not hire local physicians, nor do they include them in planning and decision-making processes.

I recently took part in a 2-day meeting of CEOs from organizations doing work in Africa. The meeting was about how we could collaborate to set goals to increase our collective impact in a particular country. The problem was there were only U.S.-based organizations at the meeting, but not one African representative. We were able to redirect the meeting toward goals of better collaboration and resource sharing between organizations, but only after we realized we were walking out the classic model of paternalism. The challenge is that everyone in the room knew better, but we still headed down that path of paternalism. We quickly recognized no discussion about collaborative goals was appropriate without our African colleagues that need to set the goals and own the process being at the table.

The provision of free, unsolicited goods and services to communities is paternalism. It assumes that those coming to serve know what is best for the population they will be visiting. Some volunteer healthcare professionals from wealthy countries sometimes exhibit beliefs or subliminal attitudes that exacerbate paternalism. Volunteers sometimes believe their training, skills, knowledge, and abilities are superior to those of local providers. In many instances this is true, but the belief itself immediately subordinates local providers. We must take care to go as learners, recognizing the dignity of our colleagues in low- and middle-income countries. This paternalistic attitude is not isolated to short-term volunteers—it is sometimes present in longer-term expatriate global health workers. We need to remember Best Practice Guideline 2, Go as Learner, Not as a Teacher. Not that there is no need for nursing educators and physician residency faculty. There is, and many of full-time CHSC staff serve in those roles in several countries. Go as Learner Not as Teacher refers more to an attitude than a role. It's about recognizing how little we know about providing care in the resource-poor context and how much we have to learn. Starting with a learners' attitude edifies our local colleagues, builds relationships, and opens paths for two-way learning.

Local providers are often more capable of providing primary care in their communities than some visiting healthcare workers from the developed world. They trained to function within resource-poor environments and are familiar with guidelines for practice for low- and middle-income countries. They are familiar with treating diseases and conditions that are foreign to visiting practitioners. They also have experience with how to access higher levels of care within their country's health system.

Paternalism also goes beyond healthcare projects; it has been a growing problem with the increase of volunteers of all kinds traveling to serve in low- and middle-income countries. The deep poverty they encounter in low- and middle-income countries often emotionally moves well-intentioned global health volunteers. Many times, this prompts them to send vast amounts of aid without considering the consequences.

The country of Haiti, with its devastating poverty and proximity to the US, is the poster country for paternalism. Haiti exemplifies how paternalism fosters dependency and disempowers the recipients of aid. It is important to pay close attention to this point because missing it could mean stripping dignity from local partners and those served by the project.

In places where global volunteers visit regularly, long-term workers report that local people rarely take ownership of their community's problems or attempt to solve them without outside assistance. Having outsiders come in to do what can be done by local people often undermines the motivation of local people to improve their quality of life. It can, and often does, contribute to a sense of helplessness in those being served.

It is difficult to understand the effect on the spirit and self-worth of a person forced to receive charity. However, on the larger scale, there is clearly a cycle of dependency that charity creates. Harvard-educated Zambian economist Dambisa Moyo, in her book *Dead Aid,* describes how the over one trillion dollars in charity that has entered Africa is likely responsible for its present continued impoverished state (Moyo, 2009). Moyo illustrates how overreliance on aid has trapped developing nations in a vicious cycle of aid dependency, corruption, and further poverty, leaving them with nothing but the "need" for more aid (Moyo, 2009). She also points out the difference between African countries that have rejected the aid route and prospered (countries like Botswana and South Africa) and others that have become aid-dependent and have seen poverty increase. This economist's view is extreme by most standards since she advocates complete withdraw of aid from the continent. However, her work points us to a profoundly important concept. All aid organizations, including those engaged in global health, need to have at least some focus on empowerment. Helping people is about encouragement, edification, and facilitating the achievement of self-sufficiency. If not well-thought-out, global health projects can make people feel incapable of meeting their own needs and indebted to our benevolence.

One of the major concerns about global health initiatives from the community development world is that they make the serious mistake of providing *relief* in situations where *development* is the appropriate intervention. The purpose of relief is to provide immediate charity in emergency or crisis situations, whereas development is about improving local self-sufficiency and capacity. Giving handouts of goods and services (even medical services) in situations that call for development can do enormous damage to development efforts. It is a simple truth found in almost any international community development textbook that providing relief in these situations impedes development and causes harm. It causes harm by undermining the capability and willingness of resource-poor communities to steward their own resources (Corbett & Fikkert, 2007).

We must exercise caution in designing and carrying out global health initiatives in cooperation with local communities and health systems. They need to initiate, control the effort, and then invite volunteers into it. Far too often it is the other way around. We create a project we think would be good for the community, invite them into it, then wonder why it failed when we leave. This is the classic mistake of small organizations and programs looking to do some good work, healthcare or otherwise. Paternalistic endeavors are why we see so many nonfunctioning water wells and empty clinic buildings around the world. The organizations never considered the projects as belonging to the community—it was theirs. Working in a community outside the direction of local health authorities is inappropriate for several reasons. We will talk more about this later. For now, it is sufficient to say, there is concern it will result in a paternalistic program that provides relief in a context where development is needed.

Empowerment manifests from asset-based approaches— dependence manifests from need-based approaches.

Have you ever done a needs assessment in a low-income community? I often ask audiences this when I'm speaking at conferences. The answer is almost always yes, and my reply is always please don't do that anymore. We need to eliminate the terminology "needs assessment" from our vocabulary. If I make a list of all the things you lack, all the deficiencies you have, all the things you need, that becomes a very disempowering place to start a relationship. It immediately causes a power shift in the relationship because it brings attention to the disparity of resources between those of us from wealthy countries and those who live in low and middle-income countries. However, if my starting place is to make a list of all the assets you have, all the capacities you have, all the resources you have—that becomes a very empowering list. This process is known as Asset Based Community Development, and it is the starting place for building programs that support human dignity and respect the professionalism of our colleagues across cultures. One of the core themes of the sphere handbook is the idea that both relief and development work are build on the foundation of existing capacities (Sphere Association, 2018). If our thinking of development practice is mature, the line between relief and development becomes less defined, because the starting place for both relief and development, including our global health work, is an asset-based approach.

The key to understanding how and why to surrender ownership and control of global health work is understanding partnership dynamics between those from wealthy countries and those in low- and middle-income countries. Deborah Ajulu, a Kenyan researcher at Oxford University, developed a set of frameworks for understanding partnerships between people in wealthy countries and people in low- and middle-income countries (Ajulu, 2013). She is the author of *Holism in Development: An African perspective on empowering communities.* She identified three types of partnerships between people in the wealthy countries of the global North and people in poor countries of the global South (Ajulu, 2013).

The first model she describes is the cow and milker. In this type of partnership, volunteers from the global North travel on an airplane to the global South. They arrive in a village in an SUV or bus, usually wearing nice clothes to do some good work. The villager in the global south immediately sees the visitor from the wealthy country as a cow that needs milking. They direct and lead the cow in the direction that will produce the most milk for them. This happens to both short-term volunteers and long-term cross-cultural workers. It can be hard to avoid.

The second partnership framework Dr. Ajulu theorized, was that of the horse and the rider (Ajulu, 2013), a model in which those in the global North travel go for a good equestrian adventure on the backs of those in the global South. They direct and guide the local partner to provide a wonderful experience based on how the expat visitor defines it. Almost all short-term global health initiatives fall into one or both of these two categories. To some extent, even large organizations fall into one of these two paradigms, because control of funding often means control of the project or program. Programs by large organizations, such as universities from wealthy countries, are often paternalistic in structure. They are planned and created by us in the global North, and then our local colleagues in the global South are invited to take part, instead of involving local partners in every step of the design, implementation, monitoring, and evaluation of a project. I will describe more about this when we get to best practice Guideline 6 that focuses on participatory design monitoring and evaluation.

During my years of serving in and studying global medical work, I have seen very few volunteer initiatives or global health service learning initiatives that do not fall into one of these two partnership models. The problem with these two types of partnerships is that they are both dysfunctional and codependent. The global South partners see the North as a revenue source, upon which they depend and will do just about anything to keep. Meanwhile, the global North partners derive a sense of purpose and meaning from serving the poor in the global South. These models often fall into place unintentionally; they do not form from some devious intent. They are just the natural way relationships develop when those operating from the higher end of Maslow's hierarchy of needs form relationships with those operating from the lower end of Maslow's hierarchy. From volunteer medical workers, to global health service-learning teams, to universities working on grant-funded research projects, most seem to end up in this trap—possibly because there is control that intrinsically comes with having financial resources, or even perceived potential for financial resources. It's the golden rule of working in poor communities: the one with the gold rules. It's hard to get beyond the one with all the resources having all the control. But we need to get past both of these dysfunctional models so we can develop healthy cross-cultural partnerships. There can be healthy cross-cultural partnerships to which we can aspire.

Dr. Ajulu describes a third model of partnership between the people in the global north and people in the global South, which she describes as a mutually transforming partnership (Ajulu, 2013). This form of partnership is extremely rare in short-term global health projects i.e., less than a few years. A mutually transforming partnership is where both sides of the collaboration learn and grow from each other, complement each other's strengths and weaknesses, and accomplish more together than either could accomplish individually. It is hard for mutually transforming partnerships to develop without the outsider living and working in the community long-term. It requires building relationships over time. It will also require many open and honest cross-cultural conversations about what constitutes healthy and unhealthy partnerships. If both sides understand these three models of global partnership and will discuss them, it is likely they can develop a truly transformational partnership. In the next chapter, we will look closer at the why behind *Best Practice Guideline 3 - Surrender Ownership and Control to the Community.*

References

Ajulu, D. (2013). *Holism in development: An African perspective on empowering communities.* Seatle: World Vision Publishing.

Corbett , S., & Fikkert, B. (2007, March 2007). *News at chalmers.org.* Retrieved November 21st, 2011, from Chalmers Center for Economic Development: http://www.chalmers.org/news/mar-2007

Moyo, D. (2009). *Dead aid: Why aid is not working and how there is a better way for Africa.* New York: Farrar, Straus and Giroux.

Chapter 11
Community Empowerment

Best Practice Guideline 5

Build Capacity

Surrender Ownership and Control of our Projects and Programs

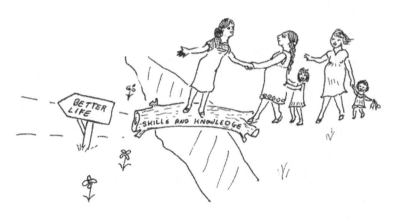

Used with permission of Hesperian Health Guides

'Empowerment is demonstrated by the quality of people's participation in the decisions and processes affecting their lives. In theory, empowerment and participation should be different sides of the same coin. In practice, much of what passes for popular participation in development & relief work is not in any way empowering to the poorest and most disadvantaged.'

Page 14, The Oxfam Handbook of Development and Relief, Deborah Eade and Suzanne Williams, 1995.

Empowerment or Disempowerment

A case study from Latin America

A pastor in Guatemala asked a partner church in North America if they could send a medical team to provide medical care in his community. The pastor knew his partner church in Vancouver had several doctors, nurses, and non-medical volunteers that would be willing to volunteer. The church sent a team in response to his request. He directed the team to three communities where they held clinics in local churches. They saw 200 patients per day for seven days in a rural area that they believed had very limited access to healthcare. However, on the second day, Dr. Hernandez, the primary healthcare provider for the area, arrived to extend his welcome to the team. His clinic was two blocks away. Later, a translator stated that Dr. Hernandez, his cousin, might have to close his clinic, because he was having difficulty making ends meet. Apparently, volunteer medical teams were coming to the area every two to three months, and each time they did, his business dropped off significantly for the weeks to follow. In addition, his office closed during the time the teams were there, as he stated,

"No one wants to go to a local doctor when they can go to a gringo doctor. Everyone knows the gringo doctors are so much better."

At church on Sunday, you run into Dr. Hernandez again and learn that he is board certified in Internal Medicine and did a fellowship in public health with the Pan American Health Organization in Washington, D.C.

(Seager & Seager, 2010)

Key Point

Volunteer global health initiatives will build confidence in the local health workers, or they will diminish it. The resulting outcome is often determined by the amount of direction and ownership that the local health system has over the global health project.

As this case study illustrates, global health initiatives can adversely affect local healthcare providers financially and can subvert their place of authority in the community. Such initiatives can also diminish confidence in the local health system and its providers, especially when those providers are community health workers (CHWs) trained by the government or local non-governmental organizations (NGOs). Even hospitals can be affected adversely by volunteer global health initiatives.

When I was in Haiti in the summer of 2010, I met with one of our facility partners. The hospital chief of staff there described serious economic hardship for their hospital after the earthquake. This facility was one of the more functional medical facilities in Haiti. Yet, as with all medical facilities, it was not sustainable without a payment model. This hardship resulted from all the free care being provided by volunteers from North America. The hospital administrator feared that the vast numbers of volunteer medical teams could close the hospital, since no one wanted to pay for care when they could get it free from visiting volunteers. I often ask doctors in the United States, "If a group of Canadian physicians came and set up a free clinic in a parking lot across the street from your practice and provided free care to all your patients, how would you feel? What if they never even acknowledged you exist except to express to your patients that they should not have to pay for any healthcare services or medication? What if all your patients thought the Canadian physicians were more capable than you and stopped taking the medication you prescribed for the new and better medications from the Canadian physicians?"

This facility in Haiti operates nine remote rural health clinics in the area, all of which provide basic community services such as immunizations for free. They welcome collaboration with foreign providers, but under their supervision and guidance. They have medical records on all their patients in all the nine communities and in the hospital. They also welcome specialty surgeons to come and provide services that are not normally available in the region. Their social service representative is adept at discerning which patients have some capacity to pay and which do not. Fees charged for surgical services based on the patient's ability to pay, and in this way the facility can use those funds to pay their staff and expenses. Visiting medical and surgical groups can improve the sustainability of medical facilities and health programs by working under their direction. Working outside their direction often unintentionally hurts them, both financially and by diminishing community confidence in their abilities, which can harm the general quality of healthcare available in the region.

Programs that engage in global health projects need to be cognizant of these potential effects. This awareness can help us develop strategies that minimize or eliminate these negative outcomes. There is a need and a place for global health initiatives, but when we design such programs, we need to understand the concepts of payment models and sustainability, or our efforts can damage the development process. We can also directly harm the projects and programs of the local health system by our efforts.

Bishop and Litch's (2000) article for the *British Medical Journal* describes their experience as co-directors of Kunde Hospital in the Mount Everest region of Nepal. They describe the vast numbers of volunteer doctors that come and hold ad hoc clinics with no thought of the fact that there may be a local health system, and with no thought of connecting with that health system.

The main challenge for Kunde Hospital is that it oversees a significant community health program which was being adversely affected by the misguided good intentions of outside volunteers. They explain how teams often set up and hand out antibiotics and medications for chronic diseases, completely oblivious to the fact that most of the patients are under their care in the local health system. They also describe the danger of worsening multi-drug-resistant tuberculosis (MDR TB) because of the extremely high number of TB patients in the Kunde TB treatment program and the confusion this often causes by giving their TB patients more and different medications. Overdoses and adverse drug interactions can become a significant danger in this kind of situation. I would like to report that this no longer happens. However, we still see these situations play out around the globe, especially in popular or unique travel destinations.

In early 2015, I was leaving Hospital Loma De Luz on the coast of Honduras after visiting Christian Health Service Corps (CHSC) staff there. I ran into a large short-term medical team unloading cases of medications and supplies about three miles from the hospital. The team had many North American doctors and nurses wearing matching t-shirts, so they were easy to spot. Loma De Luz is one of the most functional hospitals in Honduras where there are many Christian Health Service Corps physicians, nurses, and support staff. It has a great surgical department, emergency department, OB, and inpatient wards. It also has a large outpatient clinic, which provides ongoing care to the people in the area. I stopped and introduced myself and asked what communication their medical team had had with the hospital up the road. Sadly, their answer was not surprising: "What hospital?"

Since writing the first edition of this book, I have been asked repeatedly, "How can the information in this book be translated into a model that can be followed by short-term medical volunteers?" The answer is that it can't. Not if the intention is to use it to set up short-term medical initiatives disconnected from long-term work in the community.

This has become the classic story of short-term volunteerism of all kinds. In church mission trips, university global health initiatives, and service-learning programs. Everyone doing this kind of work says their goal is to impact the recipients of our care. Too often though, the end goal becomes to field a team to do some project—medical or otherwise—so they will derive a sense of accomplishment or purpose. Very few volunteers stop and ask the questions: "How do we support long-term global health work?" or "Who should we be connecting with to support their long-term efforts?"

Working at the community level is harder and more complex than working with a hospital or clinic that is actively providing care. It should be considered only in partnership with programs that have development experience and are already working in that community. This is because medical programs that give away free care in villages are functioning from a relief model in a context that calls for development.

Unfortunately, this is the way too many volunteer programs operate. This leads to the patient safety and paternalism problems discussed previously. Working in and through local health systems is the best way to eliminate most of these challenges. Partnership with health systems and hospitals eliminates most of the patient safety issues associated with short-term health initiatives.

Thinking about community-level global health initiatives is often completely foreign to most volunteers from wealthy countries. Working in communities is largely about inspiring the community to take ownership of their own health problems. For any project at the community level to be successful, the community must discover their problem and they must develop strategies to address it. If the community does not own it from the beginning, success is rare. What community development workers do is facilitate community discussion without offering solutions. Once the community has identified issues they want to address, the community facilitator can come alongside them to support the community's effort. We accomplish community facilitation through a process we call PLA or PRA, which we will discuss in more details in the next chapter. For now, what is important to know is that we term these community initiated programs "horizontal" programs, because they arise from the community members. Hospital systems and medical care programs are vertical and top-down, much like most western medical thinking. Even our community-based interventions such as immunizations are very top-down vertical programs. We will look at the idea of both vertical and horizontal models in this chapter so that you can identify the best fit for your global health initiatives.

It is essential that we realize that using strictly vertical approaches to healthcare delivery in resource-poor communities can be more harmful than helpful, especially if they provide medical care disconnected from the local health authorities. In many poor communities, everything from wealthy countries is perceived as better, sought after, and to be imitated, while old ways of tradition and caring may be thought of as something that should be left behind.

It is important to understand the difference between vertical and horizontal programs for a couple of reasons. First, from a best practice perspective, it is best that volunteers using a vertical approach should choose local partners also using a vertical approach to their work. Local community leaders, pastors, and even expatriates living in the country rarely understand that medical care could be harmful. In addition, medical volunteers rarely understand what is necessary for mutual design of healthcare programs that support patient safety and human dignity. Collaboration and integration with the healthcare services already serving the community is essential for designing global medical projects that support both patient safety and human dignity.

Vertical VS. Horizontal Programs

The Alma-Ata Declaration of 1978, discussed in chapter 6 gave rise to the idea of horizontal community-based programs connecting with vertical medical initiatives. That thinking has matured into sustainable models of healthcare and disease prevention. If your program plans to function outside hospitals in the community, then you need to invest time in learning something about horizontal community-based programs. If we do not learn, respect, and implement horizontal methods at the community level, there are a couple likely outcomes. We may leave a legacy of disempowerment and dependence on outside help and healthcare models that have proven unsustainable in resource-poor communities.

The opposite side to this is that if we do learn these methods, there is no limit to the positive impact the enormous volume of global volunteers could have on child mortality, maternal mortality, HIV/AIDS, malaria, and other communicable diseases. As healthcare providers trained in wealthy countries, we need to let go of the idea that our methods of healthcare are the only methods. There are methods global medical volunteers can use to serve and support such projects which we will review in this chapter.

Vertical Programs

These are often disease-specific, hospital-based, medically-driven programs.

Some are very effective—EPI (Expanded Program on Immunizations), Roll Back Malaria, and prevention of mother to child transmission of HIV are all examples of effective vertical programs.

They often undermine community ownership.

They are driven by outside planners and donors with outsiders deciding what is best for the community.

They are not sustainable if funding dries up or is reallocated to other priorities.

They often find success at the expense of horizontal approaches by attracting community workers from horizontal programs.

(Lankester, 2009)

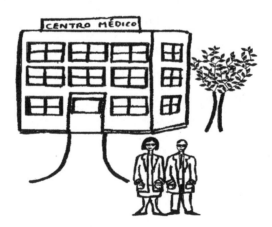

Used with permission of Hesperian Health Guides,
Burns et. al. (2012) Donde no hay doctor para mujeres

Horizontal Programs
These are community-owned and -directed programs.

They require community partnership in design and management; they are founded in mutual design that empowers the community to respond to its own health needs.

They are directed toward addressing a wide range of problems rather than a single issue.

They are prevention-focused with curative-care components.

They are volunteer operated and supported, making them very cost effective.

If there is a compensation model incorporated, it is usually modest and sustainable without outside funding.

(Lankester, 2009)

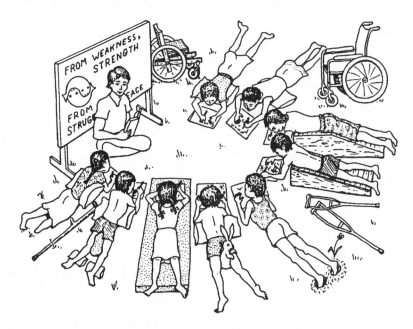

Used with permission of Hesperian Health Guides,
Werner (2009) Disabled Village Children

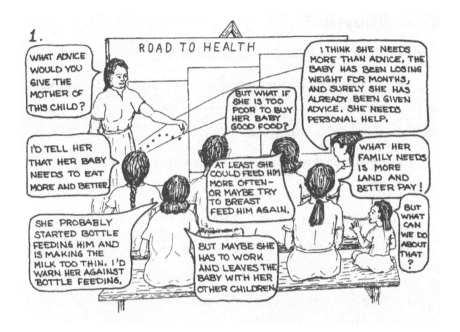

What does the Declaration of Alma-Ata have to do with global health projects?

The Alma-Ata Convention was driven primarily by the failure of vertical programs in the eradication of malaria and other such diseases in the developing world. In the 1960s, new studies emerged in community health. One book entitled Health in the Developing World by John Harland Bryant (1969), an American Christian physician, was one of the first to question the use of vertical hospital systems-based approaches in community health. Many others in public health also questioned the vertical hospital-based approach to healthcare in developing countries. Dr. Kenneth Newell's (1975) WHO report entitled "Health by the People" also questioned this model of vertical hospital-based health programs in developing countries. Ivan Illich's (1975) book Medical Nemesis: The Expropriation of Health: Ideas in Progress also helped people understand the failures of the Western medical approach in resource-poor environments (Illich, 1975). Alma-Ata directly resulted from this new way of thinking about healthcare at the community level and was an attempt to diverge from past failures to create real and lasting solutions to the health problems in developing countries.

Although the thinking that inspired it was very vertical, no one fully understood how to create quality healthcare for the poor and make it sustainable. To this day, that is a subject of much discussion. Community-based horizontal thinking drove the Alma-Ata, but those who were attempting to implement it in the beginning were not sure what that would look like. Initially, Western vertical healthcare delivery dominated attempts at implementation. Governments and NGOs built clinics in rural communities and hire medical workers to staff them. Few professional workers were interested in going to rural outlying areas. Those that went often found that their paycheck did not make the trip with them, nor did the medications promised to care for the people. There are empty, discontinued health centers in rural communities around the globe that attest to this valiant effort. There are also many abandoned hospitals that remain a testimony to the fact that vertical health systems are not sustainable without a payment model. In the same way that vertical medically focused programs are not sustainable in developed countries without a payment model, they are also not sustainable in developing countries without a payment model. There needed to be other methods for getting healthcare to the poor, and over time, these methods have emerged.

The Alma-Ata Declaration and the goal of "health for all by 2000" gave birth to new and innovative models of healthcare delivery. Health programs emerged that were horizontal, operating in the community by the people of the community serving and supporting each other in their desire to achieve better health. Alma-Ata is important because it gave birth to a movement of community-based primary health care (CBHC). The lack of understanding about CBHC is one of the primary knowledge deficits of global health programs and of the volunteers who serve in them. In retrospect, I believe my thinking about how healthcare should be done (from my North American perspective) was probably one of the most harmful aspects of my early years of working in community health. I would typically engage in one- or two-week community-based medical projects that showed a vertical form of healthcare that is not sustainable or duplicable in poor communities. Global health initiatives employ a model of healthcare delivery that has historically failed to meet the needs of resource-poor communities. If we are not fully aware of other long-term, sustainable health initiatives, we can inadvertently damage those programs.

Global health programs need to learn and understand CBHC and develop strategies to support it. Otherwise, we will continue to build dependence on our completely vertical approaches to healthcare delivery that have proven so ineffective. The best single resource for learning and understanding CBHC programs is a book entitled Setting Up Community Health Programmes: A Practical Manual for Use in Developing Countries by Dr. Ted Lankester. It is available in the US through the Hesperian Foundation (see www.hesperian.org). In Chapter 1 of this book, Dr. Lankester describes CBHC as a convergence of vertical medical programs and horizontal community-operated programs in ways that support each other.

CBHC recognizes the need for vertical hospital-based healthcare programs (Lankester, 2009). In fact, the idea is to create synergy, partnership, and integration of vertical and horizontal initiatives. There is always a need for advanced healthcare services; inpatient hospital care and safe surgery are global health priorities. The idea behind creating effective CBHC is to develop strategies in which vertical hospital-based programs are integrated with horizontal community-based programs to facilitate the achievement of better health and wholeness in communities. According to Lankester (2009), health development often occurs in three stages: Stage 1 is traditional healthcare, which uses traditional healers. He explains that at this stage, development healthcare takes place in the community according to the wishes and convenience of the people but is not usually effective (Lankester, 2009). Stage 2 is the acceptance and use of vertical Western healthcare programs. In vertical programs healthcare is provided by outsiders with specialized scientific knowledge (Lankester, 2009). In this second stage of development healthcare takes place in hospitals and clinics with the care dominated and directed by a physician or practitioner often outside the community (Lankester, 2009). The challenge is that this form of healthcare is not sustainable at the community level without an external financial support mechanism. In order to be sustainable, services and medications often involve a cost to the patient, excluding many people in need of care. In Stage 3 of the health development process, healthcare returns to the community, integrating the best of health systems-based vertical programs and community-based horizontal programs (Lankester, 2009).

Community health workers are chosen by community leaders and trained (usually by healthcare professionals) in disease prevention and basic curative care. Disease prevention and affordable healthcare then becomes available in the community from a resident of the community with referral ability to area clinics and a regional health system. Global health programs can launch or collaborate with such programs.

According to the Department of Human Resources for Health at WHO (2007), community health worker (CHW) programs are not a panacea for a weak health system, nor are they a cheap option to allow affordable access to healthcare in underserved regions. Many CHW programs have failed because of poor planning and underestimating the time and effort required to establish and sustain them (Department of Human Resources for Health at the WHO, 2007). In some areas, this has unnecessarily undermined and damaged the credibility of the CHW concept (Department of Human Resources for Health at the WHO, 2007). This being said, it is achievable for global health initiatives to start, develop, and sustain such programs. Provided the international organization returns to that community regularly to monitor, evaluate, and provide ongoing support.

There are even organizations that will provide essential lifesaving children's medications free of charge to CHW programs providing there is an organization willing to provide continued training to workers and supervision of the project. The upside to this is that healthcare workers are allowed to charge for the medications, and they receive 50% of the funds; the other 50% goes to purchase the medications from the supervising organization or health system. These funds are used by the organization to offset customs and transport charges. Medications are donated and shipped to countries free of charge, but port, customs, and transport charges are the responsibility of the receiving organization. Medications are usually supplied to area health centers for distribution to the CHWs, who then return with the medications to outlying communities. Even if CHWs are not trained to dispense medications but are only trained in general health education and to administer immunizations, there are many ways to arm them to fight disease. One example is use of artemisinin-based suppositories; putting them in the hands of community health workers to give to families with proper education has saved the lives of many children with severe malaria in developing countries. It buys enough time for them to get to a clinic or medical facility.

References

Bryant, J. H. (1969). *Health in the developing world.* Ithaca, NY: Cornell University Press.

Corbett , S., & Fikkert, B. (2007). News at chalmers.org. *Chalmers Center for Economic Development.* Retrieved from http://www.chalmers.org/news/mar-2007

Department of Human Resources for Health at the WHO. (2007). *Community health workers: What do we know about them? The state of the evidence on programmes, activities, costs and impact on health outcomes of using community health workers.* Geneva: Department of Human Resources for Health.

Illich, I. (1975). *Medical nemesis: The expropriation of health: Ideas in progress.* London: Calder & Boyars.

Lankester, T. (2009). *Setting up community health programmes.* Berkeley, CA: Hesperian.

Newell, K. (1975). *Health by the people.* Geneva: WHO Press.

Peterson, R. P., Aeschliman, G. D., Sneed, R. W., & Hurst, K. (2003). *Maximum impact short-term missions: The God commanded, repetitive deployment of swift, temporary, non-professional missionaries.* Minneapolis: STEM Press.

Chapter 12
Building Community Capacity for Healthcare

Best Practice Guideline 5
Build Capacity

5.2 Build capacity of Vertical Healthcare Programs

5.3 Build Capacity for Quality Improvement

5.4 Build Capacity Using PRA and PLA

5.5 Build Capacity Using Stakeholder Analysis and Community Assessment

A Peace Corps Story

A medical team arrived in a Honduran village in response to an invitation from a local pastor who had organized the church to be used as a clinic. The team saw patients all day and had to turn some away. One translator, a local Peace Corps Volunteer (PCV), needed a ride home, and

a friend picked her up and gave her a ride in the back of his truck—a common place to ride in the mountain villages of Central America. A young woman holding a baby wrapped in a blanket was also in the truck bed. After getting into the pickup, the PCV asked to hold the baby. The mother replied only by asking if the PCV had been working with the medical team that day. It was then that the PCV realized something was terribly wrong. The mother explained that after waiting in line all day for the doctors to see her baby; she was too far back and did not receive care. It was then that the PCV realized the baby had died. The local public health clinic was only two blocks away from the church where the medical team was serving.

(Tschiegg, personal communication, October 2005)

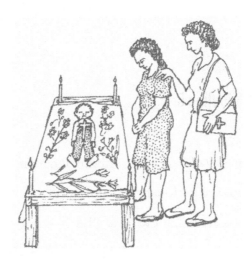

Used with permission Hesperian Health Guides,
Where There Is No Doctor Werner (2011) Illustrated by Thuman & Maxwell

5.2 Build Capacity of Vertical Healthcare Programs

This is a horrifying story about a poorly planned and poorly implemented volunteer community clinic project; not to say the baby would not have died if they received care. Many of the facilities where our organization works, 1 to 2 children die per day in peak malaria season. This is a global health reality. However, this story exemplifies the challenge of how difficult creating systems for patient safety in pop-up community clinics really is. It also shows us the dangers of doing volunteer medical work apart from existing medical work in the community.

Pairing vertical programs with vertical programs for partnering is important from both a development and a patient safety perspective. In the last chapter, we talked about two ways for volunteer global health programs to develop partnerships to serve in communities. One model is in partnership with the local health system where the local health authorities direct volunteer efforts. The other develops a partnership directly with the local community without communication with the healthcare stakeholders in the area. One common misconception held by medical volunteers is there are no healthcare services where they plan to serve. More often than not, functional healthcare services are available in the communities served by such programs. The health system and its providers in or near a community are the key stakeholder with whom volunteers need to develop a relationship. There are some regions that are so remote that healthcare services are not available; however, these are regions rarely served by international volunteers. If the global health initiative is partnering with a community so remote the population has no access, there are still healthcare stakeholders. The healthcare stakeholders could be the national ministry of health, regional health system, or rural health outposts in the region—all of which would likely love to have help from a group of volunteers to carry out primary healthcare, immunizations, disease prevention, and community health education. Even with local health system oversight, volunteers working in communities need to follow the principles outlined in this text. This text is not a comprehensive discussion of community development. It is simply an overview of key concepts related to international healthcare and development service. If you plan to work directly with communities, I strongly encourage you to seek advanced training in community development work. Colorado State University offers online certificates in Community Development through their Village Earth Program. Find out more at https://villageearth.org/. Unite for Site Global Health University also has a community development certificate program; however, it is not a facilitated course where students can interact with each other and faculty. Find out more at https://www.uniteforsight.org/global-health-university/.

Working at the Community Level requires different skills and training than working within a healthcare system. Community development training may not be essential for volunteers working under the direction of local healthcare systems or facilities. However, development training is needed for those working in a community. It means learning to mobilize the community to respond to its own problems, helping them realize they can identify and slay their lions without fully depending on outsiders. It is clear we need to exercise caution in the way we serve the poor because charity can degrade dignity and self-worth. If we do not understand this concept, we do not understand poverty. Poverty is not just a lack of money and material goods (that is the visible manifestation of poverty), but rather, at its core, poverty is a lack of self-worth. It is a pattern of limiting beliefs, reinforced by one's environment, that prevents one from reaching their potential as a human being. By stepping into poor communities without some basic understanding of poverty, we can easily reinforce existing perceptions that they must depend on outside resources. There is often a need for outside resources, but we need to recognize those resources can support or diminish dignity depending on how they are used.

Mother Teresa was asked her thoughts on the saying "Give a man a fish, feed him for a day, teach him to fish, feed him for life." Her response was profound. She reportedly said "My job is not to teach people to fish—my job is to make them strong enough to hold the fishing pole so you can teach them to fish." There is a definite place for charity and good works motivated by compassion. We should never be deterred from that aim. Understanding these concepts and thinking about them will help us mitigate the unintended consequences of our compassion and kindness. We will make mistakes when we enter and work in new communities. To Mother Teresa's point, the big picture involves both giving a fish and teaching to fish, and both are important. We achieve both aims best through healthy, mutually transformative partnerships where each partner has a role.

Speaking from the development perspective, there is a challenge with vertical programs partnering with horizontal programs because their goals are fundamentally different. Vertical programs, as discussed in the previous chapter, involve outsiders focused on providing goods and services, which can interfere with or impede community-based development initiatives. Horizontal community health initiatives are prevention-focused. If the community-based horizontal program is given complete direction over the work, it could be very effective. Global health programs seeking to develop and support community initiatives can be incredibly effective if they are willing to listen, learn, and practice participatory methods.

The potential to diminish dignity and self-worth of those in the community and offend our local healthcare colleagues is ever present. So is the potential for actual physical harm to patients that we discussed in earlier chapters. I have always said that 95% of the problems associated with volunteers in global health could be avoided by partnering medical volunteers with local medical facilities and their programs. Vertical medically focused volunteers should partner with vertical medically focused programs. The first chapters of this book discussed the patient safety issues of global initiatives. Based on the evidence presented in those chapters, we can see that vertical global health programs need to be partnered with permanent health facilities and programs, not the local church or community center. The local church and local community leaders are stakeholders that must be part of the collaboration, but the regional healthcare system must be the primary collaborating partner and keep oversight of the project.

A Donabedian structure-process-outcome framework for healthcare quality and safety (discussed in chapter 1) is achievable in global health initiatives, but only through establishing partnerships that support patient safety. Both sides of the cross-cultural relationship need to accept the responsibility for healthcare delivery and patient safety. There must also be open discussion about how to maintain patient safety between partners. According to the WHO patient safety curriculum, patients depend on several people doing the right thing and at the right time. In other words, they depend on an entire system of care, not simply on a moment of crisis care (WHO, 2010). Systems thinking is an integral part of developing patient safety-centered programs in global health (WHO, 2010). Serving alongside regional hospitals under their direction and with their priorities eliminates many of the safety issues associated with global health programs. This method provides the structure, process, and outcome monitoring needed to facilitate an adequate level of patient safety as defined by the World Health Organization (WHO World Alliance for Patient Safety, 2009).

Collaboration with all community stakeholders, including the health system, is also a standard set forth by the Joint Commission International (JCI). According to JCI Accreditation Standards for Primary Care Centers, "The primary care center, other healthcare programs and civic programs need to cooperate and partner to identify the healthcare problems and services needed within the region or community" (Joint Commission International , 2008, p. 28). The JCI Accreditation Standards for Primary Care Centers set forth several general standards for the provision of primary healthcare in low- and middle- income countries. They also define specific quality improvement standards which apply to some extent in global health programs. The WHO and UNICEF have also defined several primary care standards for developing countries. These evidence-based standards set forth by the JCI, WHO, and UNICEF are the guiding principles used as the foundation for the development of these best practice guidelines.

We have found, from both the patient safety and the development perspectives, that pairing global and local vertical healthcare delivery programs often has a positive effect on both safety and healthcare improvement, whereas pairing vertical healthcare delivery initiatives at the community level without health system collaboration usually has the opposite effect.

A Case Study of Building Capacity with Volunteers

Central American Medical Outreach (CAMO), a humanitarian organization, provides an excellent example of this type of health system development facilitated by short-term visitors. CAMO is well established in Honduras, Central America. Their vision was to assist local providers to improve health service delivery in the region, and it has been remarkably successful. Volunteer specialty physicians and surgeons who seek to serve on a short-term visit are accepted only if they make a commitment to return twice per year for five years. They are paired with a Honduran physician in a mentoring relationship and are asked to stay in email contact. They discuss cases via email and Skype and often bring in other physicians to consult on cases. Each time the mentoring physician returns, he or she does so with equipment, supplies, and new techniques and procedures.

CAMO has obtained a great deal of equipment. They also provide on-going continuing education courses such as Advanced Cardiac Life Support (ACLS) as well as having a biomedical mobile unit, which repairs medical equipment in the surrounding region. The result is that this region of Honduras has become one of the most medically advanced in all of Central America.

CAMO is an example for building medical infrastructure, improving healthcare quality, and creating self-sustaining healthcare delivery in a resource-poor community. Through their efforts, local physicians now go out to the poor, unreached areas and provide medical and dental services that were unavailable previously.

5.3 Build Capacity for Quality Improvement

CAMO provides an outstanding example of using global vertical healthcare volunteers to facilitate lasting improvements in both healthcare quality and healthcare infrastructure. From the health development perspective, partnering surgeons or specialty programs are components of very effective global health initiatives that promote and facilitate improvements in healthcare quality. If surgeons or specialty providers from wealthy countries can practice and plan regular short-term visits to a developing world medical facility, it can be very productive. Working with a local partner physician for mutual learning and skill development is valuable. The visiting physician can learn much about tropical medicine, diseases of poverty, and practicing in resource-poor settings. The visiting surgeon or specialist can impart knowledge, skills, and expertise—provided their attitude is one of mutual learning. There are also formal medical and surgical residency programs in low- and middle-income countries where physicians can plug in as visiting faculty. Many CHSC physicians serve as clinical faculty in both surgical and family practice residency programs.

As the CAMO case presentation shows, it is possible for volunteers to facilitate health system development and quality of care. One enormous concern, however, is the unintended consequences volunteers can cause if they ignore patient safety. Local providers often hold their healthcare providers from wealthy countries in high esteem. In this way, global health volunteers diminish the importance of patient safety if they do not have some focus on it. Promoting patient safety in active collaboration with local health providers can have the effect of raising quality standards, whereas dismissing it as an unnecessary regulation may have the opposite effect. The WHO Alliance for Patient Safety has invested millions of dollars and countless hours of work in programs to improve healthcare quality and patient safety in developing countries (WHO World Allience for Patient Safety, 2008). The global health community needs to be cognizant of how a lack of focus on quality and patient safety can and will affect the larger picture of health system development in developing countries. Understanding this idea of facilitating or impeding health system development is a vital concept for global health volunteers to grasp.

There is another area of concern in health system collaboration in global health initiatives, especially those focused on educational programs. Best Practice Guideline 2: *Go as Learner not As Teacher* still applies in attitude even if the official visitor role is to teach. Volunteers who serve in medical education and training need to practice humility. If you are training surgeons or other healthcare professionals, it is important to remember that many came up in school systems and programs that were academically stringent. They are highly respected in their fields and often work in extremely difficult circumstances for very low pay. They deserve our respect and admiration; using professional titles is usually an appropriate starting point, but entering these relationships with a humble servant's heart is essential. You are there to serve and support them in their work; they are not there to support you in yours.

Many years ago, we worked with a Western surgeon who acted disrespectfully, slapping the hand of a local surgeon as they were operating together. Upset with the staff, he later dumped a tray of surgical instruments. This kind of egocentric behavior has no place in any medical facility, let alone in cross-cultural programs. Global health volunteer program should edify, build up, and encourage local medical professionals. We need to pursue that end with great humility. Simply working together with the right spirit can do much to facilitate healthcare quality, even if there is no formal teaching or education program planned.

I experienced another event with a physician from the US who was with me in the Dominican Republic. He was a highly qualified MD-PhD, board certified as an emergency department physician. I had invited him to take part with a curative care component in a six-month Community Health Worker (CHW) project we organized in the Dominican Republic. This was a project we created to use global health volunteers to facilitate the sustainability of horizontal community-based healthcare programs. I had invited this physician to come along for the advance work because of his clear passion for service. I was looking for physicians who could lead such projects, and he seemed like the ideal candidate. He was brilliant, he had a passion for service, and he was willing to spend weeks at a time leading groups. It seemed like an easy decision, so I invited him to help with the coordination and setup of the medical portion of the project. I needed to see how he would interact with local medical staff and if he was humble enough to first listen, learn, and develop a sense of his environment.

At the time I was working with Mercy Ships, and we were coordinating this project before the ship visit at the local port. This meant there were still a lot of meetings with local government health officials about credentialling, visiting staff, and other logistical issues. This physician accompanied me to meetings with the local hospital director and staff. After arriving at the hospital, he immediately began teaching and directing as if he were the hospital chief of staff. He injected himself into a physician staff meeting and presented his opinion on how to manage a trauma patient in the hospital. What he did not realize was that his behaviors and actions were causing offense and demonstrated he believed the staff physicians were not capable or qualified. It was an attitude that said, *I know you are really not very good at what you do, but don't worry. I am here, and I can teach you everything you need to know. It's a good thing I showed up to rescue you.* I have great respect for this physician professionally, but he needed to learn that there are principles and practices for working cross-culturally. When we attempted to pull him out of one situation that he had injected himself into, he lost his temper and raised his voice. If he had been patient and willing to listen and learn what we had to teach him, he would have been an enormous asset to our program. This physician needed to learn PLA (Participatory Learning and Action), which is sometimes used interchangeably with PRA (Participatory Rural Appraisal). Although, I differentiate them as PLA being the practice of community facilitation, and PRA being the practice of community assessment which incorporates PLA. Both are the basis for this kind of cross-cultural interaction with all the community stakeholders.

5.4 Build Capacity Using PRA and PLA

Robert Chambers describes PRA as "a growing family of approaches, methods and behaviors to enable people to share, enhance, and analyze their knowledge of life and conditions, and to plan, act, monitor, and evaluate" (2002)(p. 3). PLA is about changing behavior and attitudes from dominating to facilitating, establishing rapport, inviting local people to teach us, respecting them, having confidence that they can do it, and handing over responsibility. It is about empowering and enabling them to map, model, diagram, list, count, estimate, rank, score, analyze, present, plan, act, monitor, and evaluate themselves, and to own the outcome (Chambers, 2002). We will discuss and more clearly define PLA and PRA in the next chapter. Before we get too deep into PLA we must look at community assessment and stakeholder analysis. Because it is the starting point for community mobilization.

5.5 Build Capacity Using Stakeholder Analysis and Community Assessment

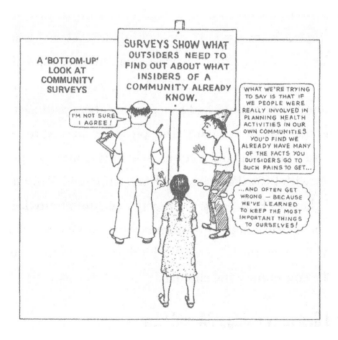

Used with permission of Hesperian Health Guides Helping Health Workers Learn Werner and Bower (2005)

We discussed facility infrastructure and site assessments for surgical initiatives in a previous chapter. This section will discuss assessment of community-level involvement in global health initiatives. Once an invitation has come from a community for a health team, community assessment is the next step. This begins with stakeholder assessment. There are four steps to this process, and they are:

1) Identify and define the characteristics of all key stakeholders.

2) Assess how the different stakeholders might affect or be affected by the project.

3) Understand the relations between stakeholders, including any potential conflicts of interest or expectations between the stakeholders.

4) Assess the capacity of different stakeholders to take part.

(World Vision, 2012)

Identifying all the stakeholders in the community is the primary goal of preliminary community assessment for global health initiatives. It is also the first step in the health project cycle, which we will discuss in more detail in the next chapter. It is normal development practice to separate stakeholders by differences within the community (e.g., gender, age, wealth, health workers, medical professionals, health volunteers). It is important to discuss openly the characteristics of all the community stakeholders (village leaders, government staff, healthcare workers and professionals). It is also important to discuss how they will be affected by the initiative the community starts.

Stakeholder analysis helps incorporate the knowledge and opinions of the people in the planning and management of the health initiatives. When entering a community for the first time to discuss potential projects, the goal should be "participatory entry," which is the foundation of mutual design. This process begins to help both the community insider and outsider development gain perspective. It is often over the course of months as the outside development practitioner works to gain persoeParticipatory entry means we should start with the local context and priorities of the people themselves (World Vision, 2012). The health situation, socioeconomic and worldview context of health, and current health initiatives should be explored together with community stakeholders once they are identified. This applies more directly to organizations than individual volunteers. However, a working knowledge of stakeholder analysis is valuable for any volunteer in global health.

Stakeholder analysis is used to identify all the stakeholders and analyze how they might take part in, affect, or be affected by the global health initiative. Stakeholder analysis is the first step in planning and designing the health project. However, it should be continued at intervals throughout the project duration to monitor, review, and evaluate the level and variance of stakeholder participation in a project. The following stakeholder matrixes were created by World Vision and can be found along with much more detailed information in the document entitled "Transformational development supplementary program resource guide on community participation" (World Vision, 2012). You can find this document for further study or community participation on the Transformational Development website at www.transformational-development.org.

Stakeholder Matrix 1

Stakeholders	Inform	Consult	Partnership	Initiate Action/ Decision Making

According to World Vision Stakeholder Matrix 1, it is more useful to conduct a stakeholder analysis on specific components or activities rather than on an entire program. This is because expected and desired participation will vary between activities (World Vision, 2012).

Stakeholder Matrix 2

	Inform	Consult	Partnership	Initiate Action/ Decision Making
Identification				
Planning				
Monitoring and Evaluation				

Matrix 2 is a more general matrix that can look at the entire project cycle. Here, instead of listing the stakeholders, the different stakeholders are placed by name in different boxes according to how stakeholders may take part at different stages of the project.

Stakeholder Matrix 3

Project Activities	Inform	Consult	Partnership	Initiate Action/ Decision Making

Matrix 3 can look at the types of participation expected by different stakeholders across a range of different project activities (World Vision, 2012, p. 9). Names of stakeholders are placed in the various boxes based on their expected participation in various activities. You can find many more tools on fostering partnership through participatory methods at www.partnerships.org.uk.

The following table includes the primary community-level assessment for evaluating any global health project site. It is an example of community assessment used by many community health organizations. The original authorship is unknown, but this form has been in use for some years. It is by no means comprehensive; it is a starting point to learn about the community. It is only an outline of key information we have used to start the community assessment process. It can be given to the individual or group who invited you to their community. For volunteers who plan to provide a primary care or dental clinic, it is very helpful in discerning what healthcare stakeholders are involved.

Preliminary Stakeholder and Community Assessment

COMMUNITY NAME:					
ADDRESS:					
TELEPHONE:					

			Yes		No
1.	Does your community have a history of self-help type projects?				
	List the projects that you are aware of, even if they were not successful:				
	a.				
	b.				
	c.				
	d.				
2.	Has your community been established for at least 10 years?				
3.	Are most of the people from one tribal group?				

4.	Is there a central meeting place in your community?				
5.	Are there definite boundaries to your community?				
6.	Is there a local dispensary within 5 km?				
7.	Does the dispensary have a mother-child health clinic?				
	(care of pregnant mothers, immunizations, family-planning services, etc.)				
8.	How far is the nearest health center?	km			
9.	How far is the nearest hospital?	km			
10.	Is public transport available?				
11.	If so, is it sufficient?				
12.	Are there any community-based healthcare activities in your community right now? If so, list them:				
	a.				
	b.				
	c.				

13.	List three of your community's problems which you think might be solved by community health empowerment:			
	a.			
	b.			
	c.			
14.	Are there other outside aid or development projects in your community right now, such as World Vision, Feed the Children, Family Plan International, UNICEF, etc.? If so, list them:			
	a.			
	b.			
	c.			
15.	Check the box that most closely describes your community:			
	NOMADIC - Almost always moving with short stays. They do not grow crops.	SEMI-NOMADIC - Moving back and forth once or twice a year. They grow crops.		
	RURAL - Agricultural. They do not	URBAN - They live close to or		

		move. They grow crops.	within a town or city.			
16.	Check the box that most closely describes the water situation in your community:					
		Almost always available.				
		Usually available but difficult to find every 3 or 4 years.				
		Difficult to find and not always available in this area.				
17.	How far must you go to obtain drinking water?	km				
18.	Check the box that most closely describes the food situation in your community:					
		Food is almost always available or easy to find or grow.				
		Food is usually available but sometimes hard to find or grow.				
		Having enough food is a constant problem.				
19.	List the common foods grown in your area:					
	a.					
	b.					
	c.					
	d.					
	e.					

20.	Would you describe any of the following social situations as a major problem in your community?						
		List any other problems in your community:					
	Alcoholism	a.					
	Prostitution	b.					
	Unemploy-ment	c.					
21.	List the major health problems in your community:						
	a.						
	b.						
	c.						
	d.						
22.	List the churches in your community:						
	a.						
	b.						
	c.						
	d.						

Once this information is obtained, we can work with local partners to ensure all the local stakeholders have been identified and contacted. They can also arrange meetings and begin the PRA processes and stakeholder analysis in the community. This is not the role of a volunteer or visitor to the country. Unless you are on the ground full-time, you cannot carry out the PRA process with the community, and definitely not in a way that would lead to the design, monitoring, and evaluation of a health program. However, it is feasible for you to use PRA in partnership with those who invited you to the community. They are your link to the community; they have the trust and established relationships. Your role as an outsider is to walk them through the PRA/PLA process. Your attendance at community meetings may be acceptable, but ideally, those meetings will be facilitated by the long-term worker in the community. There are a number of resources listed here to assist your local partners so you can learn together what this process looks like. There is one important thing you need to remember in PRA application: You will make mistakes—lots of them. Embracing them openly and learning from them in collaboration with your local partner is essential. PLA is what many have come to call PRA, and in my estimation, it is more fitting, because we learn through the project cycle together. We will talk more about PLA in the next chapter.

References

Chambers, R. (2002, January). Participation, power and social change team. Retrieved from http://www.ids.ac.uk/ids/particip

Joint Commission International. (2008). *Accreditation standards for primary care centers.* Oak Brook, IL: Joint Commission International.

The Christian Health Service Corps. (2011). *The Christian health service.* Retrieved from http://healthservicecorps.org/

WHO. (2010). Patient safety education curriculum. Retrieved from http://www.who.int/patient-safety/education/curriculum/en/index.html

WHO World Alliance for Patient Safety. (2008). *Summary of the evidence on patient safety.* Geneva: World Health Organization.

WHO World Alliance for Patient Safety. (2009). *Conceptual framework for the international classification for patient safety.* Geneva: World Health Organization.

World Vision. (2012). *Supplementary resource guide.* Retrieved from http://www.transformational-development.org/Ministry/TransDev2.nsf/ministry/

TransDev2.nsf/subsection/FCC9F534E224CAA688256F40005C38CA?editdocument

Chapter 13
Facilitating Transformation

"Promoting people's participation implies a very different way of working, different approaches, methods and expectations. A radical change in project operations, not simply the adjusting of the project planning cycle to allow for a degree of local involvement." (United Nations, 1999 ; World Vision, 2003

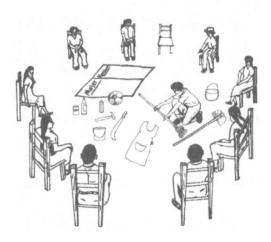

Used with permission of Hesperian Health Guides,
image library reference # 12488802

Best Practice Example:

Short-term initiatives with long-term impact

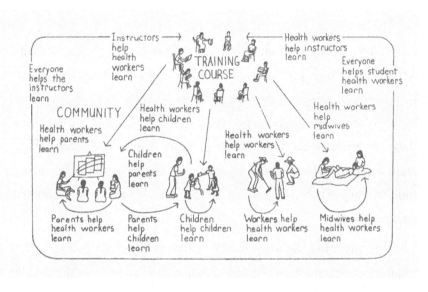

Used with permission of Hesperian Health Guides Helping Health Workers Learn
Werner and Bower (2005)

A few years back, I was approached by a physician at the Global Missions Health Conference. She had heard my wife and I speak a couple of times over previous years, which caused her to rethink how they were doing their healthcare projects. She was part of a group of physicians going once per year to the same community in Ghana to provide curative healthcare. They felt like the efforts made little or no long-term impact, and they were searching for ways to make a long-term difference in the community with which they were partnered.

After hearing us talk on facilitating health development with short-term teams, they decided on a different approach. They encouraged the community leaders and local health workers to hold a meeting, and together identify their three biggest health challenges. They then encouraged the community to develop a plan to address one of these three issues. The community determined malaria as the health problem that needed to be addressed first.

The volunteer physician group then worked to fill the gaps in the community plan providing only what was needed for the community to respond to its own problem. The next year, the physician volunteers returned to Ghana with only what the community requested. An extensive supply of donated bed nets and stacks of teaching material on malaria so the community could carry out the program they had designed. The program was nothing fancy but very impactful and empowering to the community. They planned to monitor the Malaria prevalence and compliance on return visits.

This one initiative began a partnership with the community that was mutually transforming, and many such initiatives came from this one starting place. They had discovered the secret to community development success. The community must own the problem and solution from the beginning. If the community does not own and start the project, it will never last. One technique I have seen used for this is to give the community a book called *Let's Build Our Lives Together* by Dr. Dan Fountain. It is a simple book with one line per page with illustrations that demonstrate forming a committee and brain storming problems and solutions. The better development practitioners want the community to have taken this step before they step in with the PLA facilitation techniques that will allow the committee members to unearth deeper issues. This type of community mobilization rarely happens as part of a short-term volunteer initiative. However, organizations that have a long-term presence and are working in community mobilization can incorporate volunteers in their work. This applies at the community level, and at the health system level. Recall the CAMO example from earlier where volunteers were used to improve the quality of care provided in the health system.

One thing global medical programs need to understand is that using volunteers in global health initiatives is a means, not an end. Achieving best practice in such initiatives means viewing such projects as part of a continuum of care, not as standalone healthcare projects. This means designing projects that are bigger than one healthcare group, and having groups facilitate global health initiatives that truly improve the health of a community. The challenge in this is that we need to understand community participation and the way in which it can be used to empower communities. Developing empowering partnerships and mutual design are the third and fourth standards cited by the standards of excellence in short-term missions (Collins, 2006). But what do these empowering partnerships look like in the realm of global health initiatives?

According to the United Nations Development Program's Guidebook on Participation (as cited in World Vision, 2012): "People must sit center stage and their interests be taken into consideration during the whole course of the project." This means any project or program designed to serve the poor must centralize the idea of community participation from the inception of the project to the end of the project—no exceptions.

This contradicts how most global health programs operate. The typical leader of a volunteer team goes into a community and announces that he or she would like to bring a medical team. They decide what the community needs as if they are parents caring for children. Very few communities will say no to the idea of a medical team. However, not facilitating a dialogue about community goals, and objectives can be paternalistic and disempowering. Empowering models of global health initiatives involve collaborating in ways that serve and support the community efforts to meet their own needs, usually over a period of time.

Best Practice Key Point

Global initiatives are a means to facilitate the end goal of empowering communities to improve their own health.

Creating empowering partnerships cross-culturally that are based on mutual design sounds easy, but nothing could be further from the truth. Mutual design based on community participation is one of the most difficult and complex aspects of designing and implementing global health initiatives. If done well, the end result will be a facilitated form of community participation. If done poorly, it results in forced participation and manipulation. The book *Two Ears of Corn* by Roland Bunch shows this idea of harmful, forced participation; it is a classic development book that every leader of an international program should study. Although focused on agriculture, *Two Ears of Corn* demonstrates important concepts of community development (CD) that apply to all types of community initiatives.

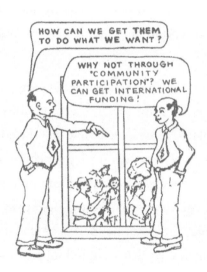

Used with permission of Hesperian Health Guides
Helping Health Workers Learn Werner and Bower (2005)

So how do we create global health initiatives that are truly based in community participation and not forced—or worse—paternalistic? The answer to this rests in PRA and PLA, which are very important models of community facilitation for anyone who works in global health projects and programs. According to Chambers (1999), "participatory learning and action" is a more accurate title for what practitioners of PRA do, but PRA is the common term used to describe participatory programming. PRA is also used by some to stand for Participatory Reflection and Action, because at the center of PRA are "self-critical awareness, personal behavior and attitudes, and engagement with action" (Chambers, 1999 p.7). When conducting PRA, it is important to remember that "we are not teachers, transferors of technology, but instead conveners, catalysts, and facilitators" (Chambers, 2002). In using participatory methods, we must learn to put our knowledge and ideas in second place; this is true from site assessment all the way to project implementation (Chambers, 2002). The goal is always to "enable local people to do their own investigations, analysis, presentations, planning, and action, to own the outcome, and to teach us, sharing their knowledge" (Chambers, 2002). We must learn to move out of the driver's seat and facilitate the community's appraisal, presentation, analysis, planning, action, monitoring, and evaluation (Chambers, 2002). You may have heard of RRA (Rapid Rural Appraisal), however, there are clear distinctions between PLA and RRA. RRA is about data collection, with the analysis done mainly by the outsider (Chambers, 2002). PRA, which is an evolved form of RRA, is meant to be empowering: a process of appraisal, analysis, and action by local people themselves (Chambers, 2002). Methods for RRA include observation and semi-structured interviews, while PRA/PLA methods are done in groups and include participatory mapping, diagraming, and making comparisons (Chambers, 2002). The following is a list of methods commonly used by PRA/PLA practitioners. Most are applicable in community gatherings as discussion facilitators, but they may or may not be applicable when working with medical professionals. The essentials of PLA are attitudes and behaviors that say, *I am here to listen and learn from you.* We need to develop what PLA practitioners call "critical self-awareness." Chambers (2002) describes the important aspects of self-awareness as embracing doubt, learning from error, and continuously trying to do better; building learning and improvement into every experience; and taking personal responsibility. This, again, is an overview of these techniques, as they appear in the World Vision supplementary resource guide on participation. They are not meant to replace formal training in participation.

PRA Tools	
Diagramming & Visualization	
Tool	**Type of Method**
Community mapping	Past, present, and future mapping to describe history and desired future. Social mapping. Resource mapping.
Drawing pictures	For "visioning" or to portray any aspect of community life.
Venn diagrams	To describe the roles/relations between institutions and people within or around a community. Also known as "chapati diagrams."
Pie charts	To estimate relative proportions (e.g., for livelihood analysis).
Daily activity profile	Describes daily patterns of activities (e.g., men/women/girls/boys).
Flow/causal diagrams	Explore cause-effect relationships (e.g., problem tree, impact flow chart).

Mobility mapping	Explores people's spatial and activity patterns and their perceptions of relative place and importance.
Mind mapping	Explores people's perceptions of different topics in relation to them.
Transect walk	To assess/map environment, land use, etc. across a community.
Seasonal calendar	Describes seasonal patterns of activities. Useful for planning.
History timeline	Explores key events in community past and/or trends on a topic over time.

(World Vision, 2012, p. 8)

PRA Tools	
Ranking and Scoring	
Tool	**Type of Method**
Wealth ranking	Explores people's perceptions of poverty and classifies households into relative poverty level. Can enhance poverty focus of projects.
Preference ranking	Expresses community opinion/preferences on a topic. Pairwise ranking.
Matrix scoring	Expresses community opinion/preferences on a topic.
Ten seed technique	Can be used to estimate relative prevalence/opinion on a variety of topics.

(World Vision, 2012, p. 8)

PRA Tools	
Verbal other	
Tool	**Type of Method**
Semi-structured interview	Used informally with all other PRA tools and/or by itself to explore a person's experiences and opinions on a particular topic.

Focus group	To explore a selected group of people's experiences/opinions on a topic.
Brainstorms	Open-ended listing of perspectives and ideas on a topic.
S.W.O.T. analysis	Helps people to consider strengths, weaknesses, opportunities, and threats of a situation/activity. Useful in planning.
Storytelling	Open-ended sharing of people's experiences on a topic.
Role play	To illustrate and communicate situations effectively.

(World Vision, 2012, p. 8)

Those engaged in community-level global health initiatives or working with community stakeholders to design a project or program need to practice participatory methods in pairs or small groups. I say this because most of the pitfalls of PLA are often personal traits that are difficult to recognize in yourself. Until you develop participatory skills from experience, it is best to have someone with you who also understands these concepts so he/she can point out when you miss the mark. Chambers, in his 1999 publication "Relaxed and participatory appraisal: Notes on practical approaches and methods," describes some common errors in the application of PLA principles, which include the following. These are things we all do at times, but when working cross-culturally, we need to be extremely cognizant of them so we can learn and grow as facilitators.

- Interrupting and interviewing people, and suggesting things to them, when they are trying to concentrate on mapping, ranking, scoring, diagramming
- Imposing "our" ideas, categories, values without realizing we are doing it, making it difficult to learn from "them" and making "them" appear and feel ignorant

- Rushing, lecturing, and interrupting instead of listening, watching, and learning

(Chambers, 1999)

One of the best ways to start the process for global health projects is to write up an outline for a project. PLA methodologies help us think through the process of guiding the community to design, monitor, and evaluate their own health project. This is not about creating a formal 10-page proposal, but it should contain some key goals and objectives set by the community and local health workers. Using PLA methods, we can help identify specific issues the community would like to address. According to Dr. Rajni Bagga (2012) of the National Institute of Health and Family Welfare in New Delhi, PLA has been shown to have a number of benefits for community health development:

1. Use and application of PLA is widespread, applicable, and considered highly useful in health programming.

2. PLA generates rapport and forces outsiders to learn, listen, and understand.

3. It provides highly accurate information: local people's knowledge of local conditions is often greater than first supposed.

4. Plans drawn up in a prescriptive manner by local people are more likely to work than plans drawn up by outsiders.

5. The participative nature of the process is a "development benefit" in itself, in terms of empowering people.

6. It is highly cost-effective.

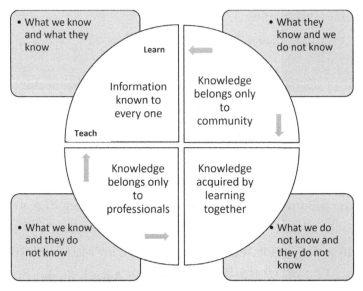

Figure 13.1. Modified from concepts presented
in a PowerPoint presentation of Dr. Rajni Bagga (2012).

Many participatory methods are to some extent whiteboard exer-
cises where the community health workers and community leaders collaborate to list all their health problems. The foreigner can encourage
such a meeting, but it is best to let the local workers and community
leaders discuss their issues and prioritize them. Be careful not to fall
into the dependency trap. It may require some steering to avoid this
becoming a Christmas list of resources the community would like your
program to bring, or things they would like to have done for them.
It is easy for our first attempts at community mobilization to unravel
quickly. They need to be steered back to community brainstorming
about how to solve their own problems. Community facilitation for
global health is about the community collaborating to list their key
health problems, prioritizing them, and then identifying their own
solutions. The PRA/PLA tools described in this chapter help facilitate

the process of identifying problems and the corresponding solutions. They also help the community discover methods for planning, implementing, and evaluating those solutions throughout the entire project cycle. Engaging the community in a project cycle is to a large extent the goal of health development programming. Easing them into the cycle and supporting them through the project cycle is something global health programs can do quite well if they understand these processes.

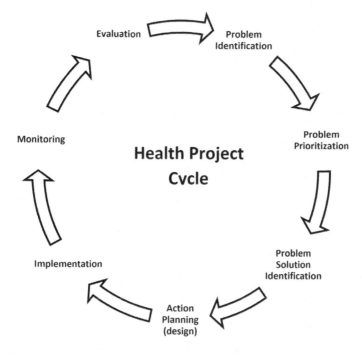

Figure 13.2. Health Project Cycle.

Based on the list created by the community and their established priorities, discussion with them can then occur on ways global volunteers may be able to assist with such projects. This may mean a number of volunteers in succession over months or years to support the program, but the key point is volunteers support the community efforts to solve their own problems. Mutual design is not deciding what is best for them and enlisting their support. Everyone in the room must participate in hopes of identifying real problems, real solutions, and the barriers to achieving those solutions. If we as outsiders contribute at all, it is to offer ways we can support local ideas, and only after all local ideas have been offered. The discussion will finally narrow to a few problems that can be addressed by the people in the community. The key items we hope to help the community bring out are geared towards creating a project-proposal outline, and they include the following:

1. A clear, direct problem statement (problem identification/prioritized by the community)

2. Project goals (exactly what change do they want to see?)

3. Project objectives (what aspects of the goal are measurable?)

4. Methods to achieve the intended goals and objectives (solution identification and planning)

5. Methods for evaluating and measuring if the objectives are achieved

With this information, you can help build a plan that utilizes global volunteers to assist in carrying it out. You can also begin to write this as a formal proposal if desired, which can attract outside funding. Community health projects are usually low cost, and volunteer project fees can typically fully fund such projects. Steps 6 and 7 in the plan or proposal process are also easy to fill in at this point if you seek to apply for outside funding.

6. Future funding if needed to sustain the program

7. Budget for the project

We turned to using health development program models to design volunteer global health initiatives after my wife and I joined Mercy

Ships, an international hospital ship organization, that also facilitates community-based projects while the ships are in port, in early 2004. We were asked to re-develop their volunteer healthcare teams program that for some unknown reason had disappeared. The ship staff was providing surgical and eye care, so it made sense that there should be medical teams providing care alongside the ships. In our naiveté, we assumed it must have been because people like us had not stepped up to the task.

When we approached the ship program staff about such projects, we realized why the healthcare teams had disappeared. The response from the ship development staff about bringing healthcare teams was something like, "Only over our cold, dead bodies will you bring a healthcare team near our community projects." I have to say, that was a bit disappointing and horribly disheartening, but they felt as most community development (CD) practitioners feel. Because of their lack of understanding, they felt healthcare teams have more potential to cause harm in the developmental context than they do to help. However, I was on a big learning curve about CD and transformational development at the time. We began to study developmental health program models and look at how global initiatives might be applied within that context. The ship's response forced us to rethink how short-term projects should and could be done. We needed to re-create them in the context of a community health developmental model.

We began to break apart the existing community health proposals and put them back together in a way that achieved the same goals and objectives but incorporated the use of global healthcare teams. The idea was to have healthcare teams serve and support the CD projects with assessment, monitoring, and evaluation. We also hoped that the groups could build the knowledge, skills, and teaching experience of the community health workers trained by the development staff.

It worked, and the healthcare teams came back to life as health development teams with a little added pre-field training for volunteers. The big change we made was using volunteers to facilitate design, monitoring, and evaluation (DME), which will be explained in greater detail in a later chapter. The key point here is that all global health programs need to have some understanding of DME and the health project cycle in order to engage the community in this process. We used DME to add the monitoring and evaluation components for community projects, which made them more desirable to funding agencies. Global health volunteers could assess and gather data for program monitoring while providing basic medical and dental services. We also found that volunteer project fees were also an excellent method for funding community-based health initiatives. These projects rarely received outside funding because they lacked the capacity to monitor and evaluate their effectiveness. However, after adding volunteers to help with monitoring and evaluation, we now had two sources of funding for such projects. The volunteer project fees and grant funding that came by using the volunteers to evaluate program effectiveness. This started as somewhat of an experiment, but the results were clear. We discovered it is possible to fit volunteers into projects in ways that empower communities to address their own health problems.

The great caution here is this could be an unintentional manipulation of the community to meet our need to feel like we have done something meaningful. Facilitating community participation is not about unduly influencing the situation so that we have a place for volunteers to go for a great "Mother Teresa" experience. It is about developing lasting, supporting relationships with communities based in respect for the dignity of all involved. We have to be mature and discerning enough to realize when attempts at facilitating community participation seem forced or manipulative/exploitative. Discussions that drift to how the community can help you and your program need to be guided back to the focus of them talking about programs they believe are needed with or without your participation.

The other great caution is we must also be willing to accept that there are some circumstances in which outside volunteer groups will always be more harmful than helpful. No matter how much medical and health need exists in that community, there may be situations in which short-term volunteers are not a good option. Communities controlled by worldviews that conflict with Western medicine is one example. Communities in which local physicians and healthcare professionals would prefer not to have volunteers visit is another. We need to respect the local healthcare providers' wishes even if community leaders would like to receive a healthcare team. We should never force global health projects and programs into places where these situations exist. In remote areas, there may be ways to incorporate small groups of instructors to train local volunteers (medical, dental, and health education) under the supervision of a missionary or aid worker in the community. These groups are usually very small and focused, and they need direct supervision by long-term personnel who fully understand both the culture of the visitors and the culture of the community. The key point is that in order to achieve best practices, global health programs need to learn and apply participatory approaches on their own or in partnership with other programs. Sometimes the difficulty is how to decide what qualifies as participatory.

There are many levels, types, and ways in which people participate in the health development process. Health development is always viewed as a continuum with different levels of independence and community ownership. The following model is commonly referred to as the community participation ladder; Sherry Arnstein originally developed it in 1969, and its use continues as a practical way of understanding participation (Arnstein, 1969). You will see many versions of it in almost every text on international CD work. The challenge is that global health programs almost always operate at the bottom of the participation ladder while most development agencies work toward the top of the ladder. This leaves a chasm between global health programs and development programs that is difficult to cross. Volunteers rarely have any perception of these concepts, and the same can often be said about the programs that coordinate and send them. In order to develop alliances and partnerships with all necessary stakeholders in a community, all global programs need to cross this divide by broadening their knowledge of community development.

Community Participation Ladder

Independent control	*Deciding together. Acting together towards mutual goals. The responsibility for plans, decision-making, outcomes, resources, and risks are equal, shared, and negotiated together.*
Partnership	*Self-management. People in communities initiate action and have ownership, power, and control over decision-making processes. They may choose to partner/consult with/inform/ manipulate others.*
Consultation	*People are consulted. Two-way communication, with opportunities for input and feedback exists, but any suggestions or concerns may or may not be taken into account in decision-making, which is still done by those with power.*
Information	*People are informed of plans, decisions, actions, and their rights and responsibilities. Mostly one-way communication, with little or no chance for feedback or potential for negotiation.*
Manipulation	*External people (e.g., those with power) decide and do things to and for the people, according to their own plans and purposes.*

(World Vision, 2012, p. 2)

Moving volunteer global health initiatives from operating at the bottom (widely considered worst or harmful practices) to the top end of the ladder (widely considered best practices) is possible. We have done this in our work, but it was not without effort. We had to change our fundamental view of volunteer initiatives from an end goal to a means goal by which we facilitate the ultimate goal of empowering communities to improve their own health. Many global programs pursue the idea of mutual design as though it is a simple concept. In reality, achieving mutual design in the context of global health initiatives means we have learned to operate at the upper levels of the community participation ladder. Community participation in a way that facilitates project design, monitoring, and evaluation by the community is the real mark of best practice. One of the "transformational development indicators" is the quality and quantity of participatory interaction. Community participation is defined as follows: "Men, women, boys, and girls perceive that they actively participate in all aspects of their community's development, with particular focus on program planning, implementation, monitoring, and evaluation" (World Vision, 2012, p. 1). Community participation is fundamental to all projects and programs that work in resource-poor communities.

The purpose of facilitating community participation is to launch a global health project mutually designed with the community and local health workers. One of the most effective uses for global health volunteers is to begin or assist health programs that will be continued by the local health community or permanent non-governmental organization health programs. The following is a list of examples that can be used to facilitate this type of community participation and collaboration. These initiatives should be carried out under the direction of local health workers and health professionals. Most present an opportunity to provide primary care if the context is appropriate but are less harmful to the health development process. They are also helpful in aligning our efforts with Sustainable Development Goal (SDG) 3. Most of the following global health models are to some extent centered on the first strategy, *The Community Health Fair*.

Community Health Fair - Working with local healthcare workers (professional and non-professional) to facilitate community health fairs is one global health strategy that can facilitate the health development process. This is a model widely utilized in the U.S. by public health departments to promote health, education, basic screenings, and primary care. These can be open to all or can be population specific, such as a child health fair or women's health fair. York (2006) identified some key concepts for designing a successful health fair based on recurring patterns within the development and implementation of these events. They are defined by the acronym HEAL:

H Helping build a sense of community

E Educating families about child health and available resources

A Advocating for the health of children and families

L Listening to the needs of families and looking for the support mechanisms within or around communities to meet the specified needs

In developing countries, support mechanisms may be limited; however, there are often more resources and support available than assumed by global volunteers. Local pastors, local health workers, local teachers, Peace Corp workers, and missionaries all have knowledge of the local community and context. Bringing all these stakeholders together for the development of initiatives helps flesh out all available resources that already exist, their distance, and the modes of transportation that can be used to access them.

Growth Monitoring and Nutrition Programs - Gathering weights, graphing data for all children, and providing nutrition education is a very helpful support initiative. Many books set forth strategies to combat malnutrition in limited-resource settings, teaching mothers how to improve nutrition despite their limited means. This basic information should be gathered in all primary care outreach models.

Ready to use therapeutic foods (RUTFs) are energy-dense, micronutrient-enriched types of peanut butter that have a nutritional value comparable to the traditional F-100 milk-based diet used in inpatient therapeutic feeding programs. Preparations such as Plumpy Nut and Nourimanba are peanut-based nutrition that can be used by global volunteers to treat children at home for mild to moderate malnutrition. Fortunately, there is no patent on peanut butter, and these foods are essentially peanut butter with vitamins, vegetable oil, and powdered milk.

Community-based Therapeutic Food for Short-term Global Health Projects

Recipe for 5 kg of Nourimanba

Ingredient using powdered/dry milk (full cream)/(skim)

Peanut paste	1250 g/1300 g
Vegetable oil	750 g/1000 g
Milk product	1500 g/1250 g
Granulated sugar	1400 g/1350 g
Formulated vitamin mix	70 g/70 g

(Partners in Health , 2010)

Assisting communities to design sustainable community-based nutrition programs is an exceptional health project in areas of high malnutrition prevalence.

It is important to remember that using RUTFs is a stopgap measure to make immediate improvement in the nutritional status of children. Nutritional counseling will also only go so far in sustaining the temporary gains. They do not change the underlying need for the availability of nutritious food. Parasite medication, RUTFs, and micronutrient supplementation will make temporary health improvements that will likely save the lives of many children, however, these gains are temporary. The focus in high malnutrition prevalence areas should be on helping communities create sustainable community-based nutrition programs.

There are a number of health initiatives that can help communities make permanent changes toward ending malnutrition. One such project is centered on moringa—specifically, providing seeds and training people to cultivate moringa in communities with high levels of malnutrition. It seems strange to some people to think about pairing agricultural projects with global health initiatives, but it is an excellent strategy to leave a legacy of hope in that community.

Moringa leaves and pods are helpful in increasing breast milk in the breastfeeding months. One tablespoon of leaf powder provides 14% of the protein, 40% of the calcium, 23% of the iron, and most of the vitamin A daily needs of a child aged one to three. It is extremely high in protein and is high in 15 vitamins and minerals (Moringa Tree, 2011). Moringa leaves contain all nine essential amino acids. The tree itself is rather slender, and it grows like a fast-growing weed, thriving in any tropical environment, humid or dry. Its branches grow to approximately 10 meters in height. It can be harvested year-round; it is often cut back annually to about 1 meter or less to allow re-growth, which produces significantly more foliage for harvesting. Nutritional content varies depending on the source cited and the moringa plant tested, but based on multiple sources, we were able to put together some averages. On average, gram-per-gram moringa leaves contain seven times more vitamin C than oranges, four times more vitamin A than carrots, four times more calcium than milk, three times more potassium than bananas, and two times more protein than yogurt (Moringa Tree, 2011). Crushed moringa seeds are also used to naturally cleanse water for drinking. They are deflocculants that, when added to water, pull solutes to the bottom of the solution. In communities in which water is drawn from rivers, this is a tremendous benefit for the community (Bruce & Kamatsu, 2010).

Moringa Oleifera for Child Survival

We have frequently paired moringa educators and trainers with global health initiatives, but the best results in any such program are to incorporate a moringa project as part of a program that develops community health workers. Moringa then becomes one aspect of their comprehensive community-based health training project. It is sometimes used as a crop through which community health workers can earn a modest income.

One such program implemented by Church World Service came alongside rural health outposts in Senegal. Healthcare workers at these rural health outposts were taught about moringa: how to grow it, dry it, and turn it into powder that could be distributed to patients for improved nutrition. Nursing mothers were taught to add a spoonful of moringa powder to their food morning, noon, and night to increase their milk production. They were also told to add moringa to all of their family meals. The health outposts that implemented this program had unbelievable results. Mothers produced more milk and children became healthier, drastically decreasing malnutrition in communities that had previously been plagued with 20% to 40% under-five mortality.

The caution in this, however, is that it is necessary in such projects to plan repeated visits to the community over a number of years, even if it is just once per year. A Mercy Ship visit to the Dominican Republic in the late 1980s illustrates that need. After setting up moringa projects in multiple communities, they left and did not follow up for several years. When they did return, they found many moringa trees all over the region, but very few people knew the tree was for food or the enormous benefits of using it.

The best community resource we have found for moringa is a book entitled *Miracle of the Moringa Tree* by Hank Bruce and Miho Kamatsu (Bruce & Kamatsu, 2010). The Educational Concerns for Hunger Organization (ECHO) (see www.echonet.org) maintains a seed bank of moringa and other such plants that can be used to support local efforts to end malnutrition in their communities.

Objective Community Health Assessments - Gathering weights and immunization data and charting growth can be invaluable for regional public health systems and local partners. This should be done as part of all primary care programs. As mentioned previously, this type of objective assessment can assist communities in identifying specific health problems and the severity of those problems so the community stakeholders can prioritize health problems, monitor progress, and evaluate existing projects.

Birth Attendant Training - This program can also fit into the model of multiple community visits. It typically requires a longer start-up but can be facilitated by supporting local healthcare professionals' efforts to implement this type of program. It is also a good add-on to already functioning community-based healthcare (CBHC) initiatives.

Prenatal Care and Infant Care Classes - This is also a much-needed program in most areas. These classes can be done as part of a health fair or as a program such as birth attendant training. Such classes are simple and have been shown to decrease infant mortality. Again, it is always best to have this kind of teaching done by community members rather than outsiders. If outsiders are doing this kind of teaching through a translator, then the focus should be on building the translator's knowledge so he or she becomes the lead in teaching the class and the outsider's role becomes one of support.

Child Immunization Programs - These can make a lasting difference in communities and save lives. Immunizations are often provided free to health centers, however, maintaining refrigeration to the end point of administration (referred to as the "cold chain") is often the biggest challenge. Collaborating with local health workers and systems to facilitate immunizations in hard-to-reach areas without refrigeration is an extraordinary service global teams can provide. Immunization programs must be under the authority of the local health system and directed by local CHWs and healthcare professionals.

IMCI Training for Local Medical Staff and CHWs - Integrated Management of Childhood Illness (IMCI) in its entirety is an 11-day case management seminar with half of each day utilizing the information in a clinical setting by seeing patients. This training is highly sought after in developing countries, and it offers a tremendous opportunity to empower both the local health professionals and the local community. The computer-based training modules developed by USAID have proven to be effective in raising the quality of healthcare services to children in developing countries (Tavrow, Rukyalekere,

Maganda, Ndeezi, Sebina-Zziwa, & Knebel, 2002). See the Christian Health Service Corps (2011) website (www.healthservicecoprs.org) for a free copy of this computer-based training program.

Palliative Care Training (PCT) Program - Preparing and training those caring for patients who are dying of HIV/AIDS is an exceptional nursing outreach program. This is a much needed program in many areas of the world. It involves training local church members in how to care for the physical and spiritual needs of those infected and dying when they are no longer able to care for themselves. This is a program that can be conducted easily by a global team with the help of a local missionary.

References

Arnstein, S. (1969). A Ladder of Citizen Participation. *Journal of the American Institute of Planners* , *35*, 216-224.

Bagga, R. (2012). *www.indmedica.com/.../ppt/participatory_rapid_appraisal_dr_bagga.ppt* . Retrieved 24 2012, February , from www.indmedica.com/: www.indmedica.com/.../ppt/participatory_rapid_appraisal_dr_bagga.ppt

Bruce, H., & Kamatsu, M. (2010). *Miricle of the moringa tree*. Rio Rancho New Mexico: Pedals & Pages Press.

Chambers, R. (1999). *Relaxed and participatory appraisal notes on practical approaches and methods*. Brighton UK: Institute for Development Studies at Sussex University.

Chambers, R. (2002, January). Retrieved February 15, 2012, from Institute of Development Studies at University of Sussex : http://www.ids.ac.uk/ids/particip

Collins, J. (2006). Standards of excellence in short-term missions. *Common Ground Journal,* 10–16.

Eade, D., & Williams, S. (1995). *The Oxfam Handbook of Development and Relief.* Oxford: Oxfam Publishing.

Moringa Tree. (2011). Retrieved January 2, 2012, from Trees for Life International : http://www.treesforlife.org/our-work/our-initiatives/moringa

Partners in Health . (2010). *Preparation_of_suggested_products_for_pediatric_malnutrition.pdf.* Retrieved June 10, 2010, from http://model.pih.org:

http://model.pih.org/files/Preparation_of_suggested_products_for_pediatric_malnutrition.pdf

Tavrow, P., Rukyalekere, A., Maganda, A., Ndeezi, G., Sebina-Zziwa, A., & Knebel, E. (2002). *A comparison of computer based and standard training in the Integrated Management of Childhood Illness in Uganda.* Washington D.C.: USDAID and University Reseach Quality Assurance Project.

York, K. (2006). Designing a child health fair. *Nursing BC, 38*(5), 17-18.

World Vision. (2012). *Supplementary Resource Guide.* Retrieved February 10th, 2012, from www.transformational-development.org: http://www.transformational-development.org/Ministry/TransDev2.nsf/ministry/TransDev2.nsf/subsection/FCC9F534E224CAA688256F40005C38CA?editdocument

Community Development Resources

Colorado State University's Village Earth program offers certificates in community development online (see http://villageearth.org/).

Community Tool Box is a comprehensive compilation of tools presently available to help your program collaborate using these empowering methods (see http://ctb.ku.edu/en/default.aspx).

Educational Concerns for Hunger Organization (ECHO) (see www.echonet.org).

The Hesperian resources are excellent resources for community collaboration and participation. Hesperian also has a section of their site where healthcare workers can construct their own health education handouts with regionally appropriate images. There are a number of existing handout templates you can customize using material from the books and image libraries (see www.hesperian.org).

ELDIS is an information/gateway site for community development materials and resources (see www.eldis.org).

Institute for Development Studies (IDS), University of Sussex, UK, is the home of participation guru Robert Chambers, a participation department, and the "Pathways to Participation" project (see www.ids.ac.uk).

Participatory Mapping Guide https://communityscience.com/wp-content/uploads/2021/04/AssetMappingToolkit.pdf

Practical Action has many community development and participation resources posted on their website (see http://practicalaction.org/).

The Institute of Social Studies in the Hague (see www.iss.nl)

The Guide to Effective Participation, by David Wilcox (1994), is available online and is an exceptional resource. It provides a theoretical framework for partnering and an A–Z dictionary with participation tools and techniques (see www.partnerships.org.uk/guide).

Books and Other Resources

Community Participation and Holistic Development' Sam Voorhies, in 'Serving the Poor in Africa MARC, 1996.

Power and Participatory Development: Theory and Practice Niki Nelson and Susan Wright, 1995

The Ten Seed Technique Ravi Jayakaran, World Vision China, 2002.

Trees for Life International has a significant number of moringa resources posted on their website. (see www.treesforlife.org/).

Walking with the Poor', Bryant Myers, 1999, World Vision / Orbis books.

Whose Reality Counts? Putting the First Last' Robert Chambers, 1997

'Participatory Learning and Action – A Trainers Guide' Jules N. Pretty, Irene Guijt, John Thompson and Ian Scoones, IIED, 1995 (www.iied.org)

Tools for Community Participation' Lyra Srinivasan, Prowwess/UNDP, World Bank Water and Sanitation Program, Washington DC.

Community Participation and Holistic Development' Sam Voorhies, in 'Serving the Poor in Africa MARC, 1996.

Chapter 14
Best Practice Guideline 6

Design, Monitor, and Evaluate Using Participatory Methods

6.3. Use results-oriented methods

6.4. Use participatory design, monitoring, and evaluation

6.5. Use participatory DME for vertical healthcare delivery projects

Patient Safety Guideline 6
Design, Monitor, and Evaluate Using Participatory Methods

In order to understand participatory design, monitoring, and evaluation (DME), we must think of it as a continuous process of improvement (or, as I like to define it, a continuous process of development) we apply to ourselves, our organizations, our processes, and our programs. DME's principles are transformative for any organization or program that commits to applying them. This chapter is an overview of DME concepts, though it is far from a comprehensive resource on this subject. There are many DME training resources available to be used as templates to help us understand health development programming. We will focus on three DME resources in this chapter, the first of which was developed specifically for participatory development programming: the World Vision LEAP program. LEAP stands for Learning through Evaluation, Accountability, and Planning. It is an excellent model that effectively demonstrates what this process can and should look like. Much can be learned about participatory DME from the LEAP training manual and supporting materials, which are available by searching for "DME" on the World Vision website. (https://www.wvi.org/sites/default/files/LEAP_2nd_Edition_0.pdf).

Table 11.1 The LEAP System

Source: World Vision LEAP training manual

Learning	Change in thinking and action through reflection on sound information about present and past experiences.
Evaluation	Systematically and objectively assessing the relevance, performance, and success (or lack thereof) of ongoing and completed programs and projects. This is done by comparing available data, monitoring implementation, and conducting planned periodic evaluations.
Accountability	Demonstrating responsibility to provide evidence to all partners that a project has been carried out according to the agreed design.
Planning	Identifying and scheduling adequate resources for activities that logically lead to outputs, outcomes, and goals. Working with management to link program and project plans to national and regional strategies.

(World Vision International, LEAP Team, 2007)

"LEAP is a living framework for systematic learning that promotes quality, accountability, and professionalism in programming <u>with communities</u>. Its implementation builds competence and confidence and models prospective learning" (World Vision International, LEAP Team, 2007).

Another exceptional resource, the United Nations Population Fund (UNFPA)'has created several toolkits for paticipatory health programs. The acronym UNFPA is a remnant of this United Nat"ons department's former name, United Nations Fund for Population Activities. This organization is dedicated to helping women worldwide have healthy pregnancies and deliveries, as well as to prevent sexual violence and to assist survivors of sexual violence. These toolkits were composed around a series of subject areas in population health for low- and middle-income countries (https://www.unfpa.org/). Another excellent DME resource is the United Nations Development Program's (1997) online handbook entitled, "Results-oriented monitoring and evaluation: A handbook for program managers" (see http://web.undp.org/evaluation/documents/mae-toc.htm).

Results Oriented Programs

Achieving alignment with Sustainable Development Goals in health means changing the ends on which we focus. It means moving from activity-oriented initiatives to results-oriented initiatives, which means learning the DME process. Making the shift in our thinking from activity-oriented projects to results-oriented programs can help us avoid providing relief in situations where development is the appropriate intervention. Relief projects are a common outcome of volunteer projects since their goals are often activity-focused, but rarely about supporting the community's initiatives for change or transformation. Global health activities in which volunteers can take part are a means—the activities are not the end goal. The need to change the way we view global medical initiatives is important to understand. This will allow us to move activity-focused projects to results-oriented programs that help produce lasting change.

To understand this change in thought process, it is necessary to differentiate projects and programs. We define a ***project*** as a time-specific intervention with established objectives and an established schedule, and from the development perspective, it is considered a collection of one or more activities usually involving a single sector. Most volunteer global health initiatives fall into the project category. A ***program*** is considered a time-specific intervention that consists of one or more projects that coordinate to achieve a desired program goal or outcome. From the development perspective, programs are often multi-sector, such as health, sanitation, agriculture, etc., requiring a multi-disciplinary approach (World Vision International, LEAP Team, 2007). In the construct of global health initiatives, we alter these definitions slightly. The use of DME helps us understand that each global health project is part of a continuum (or program) meant to improve the health of a community. Each global health project should constitute one part of a larger community-owned program.

A health program may be multi-disciplinary or focused on a single discipline, but there are usually multiple volunteer initiatives united by common specified goals with measurable objectives. In global health initiatives, many volunteer projects are used to support the goals and objectives of a program developed by, or in partnership with, community stakeholders. Global health projects that comprise larger programs can include both vertical and horizontal community health initiatives—sometimes at the same time, sometimes at different times. One example would be a dental team that provides dental services and at the same time teaches basic dentistry to local community health workers, nurses, or physicians, but as part of an initiative to increase emergency dental services in a specific region. Another example is a primary healthcare team that provides healthcare according to WHO standards, while focusing on building the knowledge and skills of local community health workers—again as part of a strategic program directed by the regional health system to improve health worker skills. Project goals may vary, such as volunteers working to provide surgical services not normally available while bringing needed medications, equipment, and supplies to the hospital.

Unintended Consequences of Good Development Practice

It is important to recognize the potential for unintended consequences, even when development is done well. For example, in Haiti, a group of development practitioners used PRA/PLA methods to develop a farmers cooperative that worked together and supported each other in rice farming. The cooperative came up with an idea of increasing rice crop yields by building a dam on the river. The farmer's plan was to keep the fields flooded longer so they could get a second rice harvest each year. They initially attempted building a river dam with no outside engineering help; sadly the first attempt failed, and the dam collapsed. The farmers cooperative raised enough funds to purchase supplies a second time, and an engineering firm stepped up to provide needed design expertise. The second time, the farmers were successful in building a dam that achieved their goal of keeping their fields flooded for a year-round growing season. Several communities in the region reaped both economic benefits and the health benefits of the increased food supply. In this context, the farmers cooperative was the program and the dam initiative was the project. The unintended consequence was by extending the length of time the fields were flooded, it increased malaria prevalence in the area. This region now has one of the highest malaria prevalence's in the western hemisphere, rivaling many African countries. So even when there is a good project design that leads us to a desired outcome, we must do our best to forecast inevitable unintended outcomes. The stakeholder analysis outlined in the previous chapter helps us identify some potential unintended outcomes.

Defining Outcomes in Global Health

How do we define results in terms of global health initiatives? The same as we do in any other programmatic approaches to problem solving. A result is a describable or measurable change in state that is derived from a cause-and-effect relationship (UNFPA, 2004). The project cycle starts with problem identification, and the result we hope to generate by entering that cycle. Each project cycle addresses an identified problem with the hope of achieving specific goals and objectives. If we cannot meet specified goals, we reevaluate, change the approach, and continue the cycle.

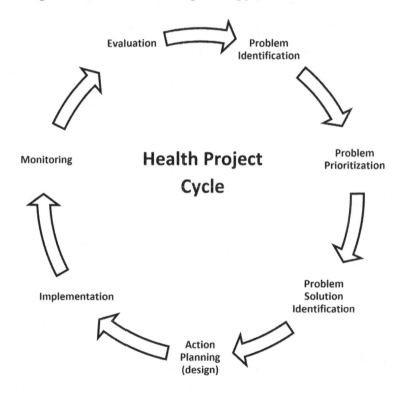

In development programming, we divide results (which we hope are solutions to the identified problems) into three categories, which include the following.

Outputs - Products and services that result from the completion of activities within a development intervention (UNFPA, 2004). These are low-level measurable results that are the end point for evaluation of most volunteer projects. This is because we can establish outputs with numbers, which are easily identified. Examples may be the number of surgeries, the number of dental procedures, the number of community health workers trained, the number of midwives trained, or the number of moringa trees planted.

Outcomes - The intended or achieved short- and medium-term effects of an intervention's outputs, usually requiring the collective effort of partners. Outcomes represent changes in development conditions, which occur between the completion of outputs and the achievement of impact (UNFPA, 2004). When we assess the outputs from an individual project, we are looking to see if they are bringing us closer to the program goals.

Impacts - Positive and negative long-term effects on identifiable population groups produced by a development intervention—directly or indirectly, intended or unintended. These effects can be economic, socio-cultural, institutional, environmental, technological, or of other types (UNFPA, 2004). We can assess the impact of both projects and programs, however, we usually measure impact at the program level. Did we facilitate the desired change?

Participatory Program Design

There are three primary steps to program design, and they include defining planned outputs, identifying the best indicators (what to monitor), and identifying means of verification (MOVs) (what and how to evaluate).

- Step 1: Define the planned outputs (goals and objectives)
- Step 2: Identify the best indicator or cluster of indicators and the performance targets to track each output
- Step 3: Identify the MOVs, timing, and reporting responsibility (UNFPA, 2004)

Define the planned outputs (goals and objectives)

Program design is a process that starts with solution identification and works backwards to action planning. This means after goals are identified, objectives are defined, and then activities are developed to meet the objectives. This is in contrast to beginning with what activities it will carry out. Program design is really designing an action plan to address various problems. This process includes laying out goals, objectives, and indicators that measure whether the objectives are being met. It also means designing methods that will address the identified problems, as well as the methods to monitor the indicators and ways to evaluate the effectiveness of the programs. Goal statements are broad, general statements of the desired outcome; objectives are specific quantifications of goal statements.

The following summary has examples of both goal and objective statements and a global health program summary that was designed with PRA/PLA methods. There are many forms of this type of initiative, but the basic principles that create such programs are the same. Participation is the foundation of all program design—they involve several projects united by common goals and objectives; there are indicators used for measuring the objectives; and there is a planned method to monitor and evaluate the community impact.

Identify the best indicator or cluster of indicators and the performance targets to track each output

Indicators can be developed from scratch, but whenever possible, we recommend using established WHO indicators. They create programs that are both better aligned with Sustainable Development Goals and with funding sources. When designing indicators to measure whether our stated objectives are being met, we must understand that there are several types of indicators. These are primarily qualitative, quantitative, and efficiency indicators. Quantitative indicators are statistical measures, such as numbers, percentages, rates, and ratios. Qualitative indicators or targets include descriptive assessments or goals related to compliance, quality, extent, or level. Efficiency indicators or targets are unit cost measures such as cost per client treated, student, school, etc. (UNFPA, 2004).

In 1998, the USAID Center for Development Information and Evaluation produced a document entitled "Performance monitoring and evaluation tips: Guidelines for indicator and data quality." This document summarizes the key aspects of program monitoring and evaluation and the standards for the evaluation of indicators. These standards for indicator evaluation are known as DOPA (Direct, Objective, Practical, and Adequate) or the DOPA criteria.

Direct

A performance indicator is direct if it closely tracks the result it is intended to measure. Indicators should be widely accepted for use by specialists in a relevant subject area. There is a strong preference for established WHO indicators.

Objective

An indicator is objective if it is unambiguous about what is being measured and what data are being collected. Objective indicators have clear operational definitions that are independent of the person conducting the measurement; that is, different individuals would collect data for an objective indicator using the same indicator definition.

Practical

A practical indicator is one for which data can be collected on a timely basis and at a reasonable cost. Performance indicators should 1) provide data to managers at a cost that is reasonable and appropriate, as compared with the management utility of the data; 2) have data available on a frequent enough basis to inform regular program-management decisions; and 3) have data available that are current enough to be useful in decision-making.

Adequate

The number of indicators tracked for a given result should be the minimum necessary to ensure that progress toward the result is sufficiently captured. There is no correct number of indicators. Rather, the number of indicators required to adequately measure a result depends on 1) the complexity of the result being measured, 2) the amount of information needed to make reasonably confident decisions, and 3) the level of resources available for monitoring performance. An objective focusing on improved maternal health, for example, may require two or three indicators to capture the various and constituent aspects of maternal health. It is uncommon to need more than three indicators to effectively track a result.

(USAID, 1998)

Identify the Means of Verification (MOVs), timing and reporting responsibility

When developing indicators for community-based global health initiatives, it is important to remember that a group of volunteers can assess an entire community. They can provide information about malnutrition and disease prevalence and a snapshot of the baseline health status of a community and monitor the effectiveness of efforts. Several community health monitoring targets have been set forth by the WHO. Most of the health assessment targets established by the WHO are directed toward SGD 3. The following are a few examples of WHO community-level indicators related to SGD 3. These indicators are presented as an example, but they are what we have used in the past for community IMCI effectiveness. Note true indicators have numerator and denominator components and track improvements in population health.

1) Proportion of infants age less than 6 months who were exclusively breastfed in the last 24 hours

   Numerator: Number of infants aged less than 6 months (less than 180 days) who were exclusively breastfed in the last 24 hours.

   Denominator: Number of infants aged less than 6 months (less than 180 days) assessed.

2) Proportion of infants aged 6–9 months receiving breast milk and complementary foods

Numerator: Number of infants aged 6–9 months who received breast milk and complementary foods in the last 24 hours.

Denominator: Number of infants aged 6–9 months assessed.

3) Proportion of children who are below the median weight for age according to the WHO/NCHS reference population

Numerator: Number of children under 2 years of age whose weight is below -2SD from the median weight of the WHO/NCHS reference population for their age.

Denominator: Number of children under 2 years of age assessed.

4) Proportion of children aged 12–23 months vaccinated against measles before 12 months of age.

Numerator: Number of children aged 12–23 months vaccinated against measles before 12 months of age

Denominator: Number of children aged 12–23 months assessed.

5) Proportion of children who sleep under insecticide-treated nets in malaria risk areas

Numerator: Number of children who slept under an insecticide-treated net the previous night

Denominator: Number of children assessed.

6) Proportion of children with fever who received an appropriate antimalarial treatment (in malaria risk areas)

Numerator: Number of children who were reported to have had fever in the previous two weeks and were treated with a locally recommended antimalarial.

Denominator: Number of children assessed who were reported to have had fever in the previous two weeks.

7) Proportion of sick children for whom the caretaker offered increased fluids and continued feeding

Numerator: Number of children who were reportedly sick in the previous two weeks and for whom the caretaker offered increased fluids and the same amount of or more food.

Denominator: Number of children assessed who were reportedly sick in the previous two weeks.

8) Proportion of caretakers who know at least two signs for seeking care immediately

Numerator: Number of caretakers of children who know at least 2 of the following signs for seeking care immediately: child not able to drink or breastfeed, child becomes sicker despite home care, child develops a fever (in malaria risk areas or if child aged less than 2 months), child has fast breathing, child has difficulty breathing, child has blood in stool, child is drinking poorly. **Denominator:** Number of caretakers of children surveyed.

Identify the Means of Verification (MOVs), timing, and reporting responsibility

Identify the MOVs, timing, and reporting responsibility refers to when and how indicators will be monitored and evaluated. In participatory programming, we assess all community stakeholders to gauge respective levels of participation. Some stakeholders will become full partners who assume the responsibility for monitoring and evaluation. In the design process, monitoring and evaluation responsibilities are agreed upon by all partners, and the specific MOVs are described. MOVs can be survey tools or objective assessments, such as weights, heights, or the prevalence of a specific disease in children.

What else makes up a good program design?

We have discussed goals and objectives, indicators, and MOVs; however, there are other aspects that constitute a good program design. A good program design provides a framework that facilitates the implementation, monitoring, and evaluation at each phase. According to UNFPA (2004), there are eight specific points that make up a good program design.

Creating effective program designs

1. ***Outputs, outcomes, and impact (the results):*** *Are they clearly stated, describing solutions to identified problems and needs?*

2. ***Inputs and strategies:*** *Are they identified, and are they realistic, appropriate, and adequate to achieve the results?*

3. ***Indicators:*** *Are they direct, objective, practical, and adequate (DOPA)? Is responsibility for tracking them clearly identified?*

4. ***External factors and risks:*** *Have factors external to the program that could affect implementation been identified, and have the assumptions about such risk factors been validated?*

5. ***Execution, implementation, monitoring, and evaluation responsibilities:*** *Have they been clearly identified?*

6. **Gender sensitivity:** *Does the program design address the prevailing gender situation? Are the expected gender-related changes adequately described in the outputs? Are the identified gender indicators adequate?*

7. **Capacity building:** *Does the program include strategies to promote capacity building?*

8. **Program approach:**

   1. *In the case of a program evaluation, does the design clearly establish linkages among programmes components?*

   2. *In the case of a program component evaluation, are linkages among its interventions clearly established to ensure synergy in achievement of program components results?*

   Source: Program manager's planning and evaluation tool kit: Tool number 6 (identifying indicators) (UNFPA, 2004)

Below, I summarize a program design that incorporates global health volunteers as an integral part of a program that was developed using participatory methods. This type of health program design includes monitoring and evaluation as fundamental to the design process. I am including it to help you visualize the three steps of defining outputs, identifying indicators, and identifying how those indicators will monitor and evaluate progress toward the program goals. It uses the WHO/UNICEF child health indicators previously listed.

This example program design is based on collaborating with local volunteer health workers and supported by a series of health fairs staffed by global health volunteers supplemental health education and pediatric primary care. Medical treatment is provided to children in need according to WHO/UNICEF guidelines. All children will be given parasite prophylaxis and Vitamin A supplementation and will be weighed, measured, and graphed at each health fair by local health workers at specified interviews. Based on assessment data collected, educational strategies and messages will be changed to meet identified needs in the community. It is based on the indicators listed previously in this chapter.

Target Population: Haitian children, age 0-5, living in two rural communities.

Health Problem: High incidence of malnutrition and mortality in children 0-5 in the target areas.

Project Goal: Identify, track, and reduce childhood disease and malnutrition prevalence in target communities.

Objective: *By December 2025 reduce by one half the severity and prevalence of all forms of malnutrition and childhood diseases in children 0 - 5 in the target communities.*

Indicators to be assessed continuously and at each health fair:

- Proportion of infants aged less than 4 months who were exclusively breastfed in the last 24 hours

- Proportion of infants aged 6-9 months receiving breast milk and complementary foods

- Proportion of children aged 12-15 months receiving breast milk

- Proportion of children who are below - 2 SD from the median weight for age of the WHO/NCHS reference population

- Proportion of children aged 6-9 months with a hemoglobin level below 11.0 g/dl4

- Proportion of children who sleep under insecticide-impregnated bed nets (in malaria risk areas)

- Proportion of children aged 12-23 months vaccinated against measles before 12 months of age

- Proportion of children aged 12-23 months who received a high dose (amount to be defined locally) of vitamin A in the last 6 months (in areas with a vitamin A supplementation policy)

- Proportion of ill children for whom the caretaker offered increased fluids and continued feeding

- Proportion of children with fever who received an appropriate antimalarial (in malaria risk areas)

- Proportion of caretakers who know at least two of five key signs for care seeking

Methods: 1) Global health volunteer teams will visit each community every six months and conduct a health fair in each community. One team will come every six months and spend 2 to 3 days in each community reinforcing health education and providing basic primary care to children and their mothers. 2) Parasite medication, vitamin A, and other micronutrient supplementation will be given every six months. 3) Growth monitoring will be continued bi-monthly by community health workers. 4) Community-based nutritional education programs will be held during and between health fairs. 5) Moringa education, planting, and cultivation will be part of each health fair. 6) RUTF will be used as a community-based malnutrition intervention.

Project Budget Summary				Total Project Duration: Five Years
Projected 10-Year Program Cost & Request		Request		Year 1's focus will be on training clinic staff and volunteer health workers in IMCI and CHE and achieving baseline-objective community assessments.
Project Cost				
G&A @ %				
Total Projected Costs				Years 2 through 5 will focus on serving and supporting local staff and volunteer workers and monitoring program effectiveness.
Volunteer Project Donations				

Treatment, Prevention, and Educational Interventions for Child Survival	
The WHO recommends five general prevention countries.	The WHO recommends four general educational interventions in developing countries.
1. Immunizations	1. Care Seeking Behaviors of parents (when to seek care)
2. Parasite Prophylaxis	
3. Vitamin A Supplementation	2. Nutrition (maternal and child)
4. Zinc Supplementation	3. Home management of diarrhea and dehydration
5. Iron Supplementation	4. Malaria Prevention, where appropriate (Maternal and Child).

Participatory monitoring and evaluation

It is important to understand both monitoring and evaluation as integral components to all global health initiatives. This may be as simple as establishing and maintaining documentation of follow-up care of surgical patients. Measuring if an intended change has occurred as a result of activities may be more complex. There is a difference between monitoring and evaluation that should be understood.

Monitoring continuously tracks performance against what was planned by collecting and analyzing data on the indicators established for monitoring and evaluation purposes (UNFPA, 2004). It provides ongoing feedback on progress being made toward achieving the desired results. It also identifies changes that may be needed in the methods to achieve the desired objectives. Monitoring tracks and compares program methods to documented changes in the target population.

Evaluation is a periodic, in-depth analysis of program performance. It relies on data generated through monitoring activities and information obtained from other sources (e.g., studies, research, in-depth interviews, focus group discussions, surveys, etc.). According to UNFPA (2004), evaluation is a time-bound exercise that attempts to assess systematically and objectively the relevance, performance, and success (or the lack thereof) of ongoing and completed programs. It is often (but not always) conducted with the assistance of external evaluators. Evaluation is commonly directed at determining the relevance, validity of design, efficiency, effectiveness, impact, and sustainability of a program (UNFPA, 2004).

Monitoring	Evaluation
Continuous	*Periodic: at important milestones such as the mid-term of program implementation, at the end, or a substantial period after program conclusion*
Keeps track, oversight; analyzes and documents progress	*In-depth analysis; compares planned with actual achievements*
Focuses on inputs, activities, outputs, implementation processes, continued relevance, and likely results at outcome level	*Focuses on outputs in relation to inputs, results in relation to cost, processes used to achieve results, overall relevance, impact, and sustainability*

Answers what activities were implemented and results achieved	*Answers why and how results were achieved; contributes to building theories and models for change*
Alerts managers to problems and provides options for corrective actions	*Provides managers with strategy and policy options*
Self-assessment by program managers, supervisors, community stakeholders, and donors	*Internal and/or external analysis by program managers, supervisors, community stakeholders, donors, and/or external evaluators*

(UNFPA, 2004)

There are four generations of evaluation; the first emerged in the 1900s and was associated with scientific measurement (Estrella & Gvanta, 1997). The next generation gave birth to program evaluation and was focused on description (Estrella & Gvanta, 1997). This second generation was very much related to performance and activity evaluation (Estrella & Gvanta, 1997). The third generation of evaluation shifted from activity and performance evaluation to results evaluation. The fourth and last generation of evaluation is where we are today, and it is grounded in stakeholder participation (Estrella & Gvanta, 1997). It considers the diversity of views, ownership claims, and economic stratification of stakeholders' consensus and opposing points of view.

This fourth generation of evaluation differs significantly from previous generations. Essentially, the differences are those that exist between conventional monitoring and evaluation and participatory monitoring and evaluation. These differences are delineated in Institute for Development Studies (IDS)"working paper number 70 entitled "Who counts reality: Participatory monitoring and evaluation" by Estrella and Gvanta (1997). The paper is a comprehensive literature review of participatory monitoring and evaluation and recognizes, in the title and text, Robert Chambers' book entitled *Whose reality counts: Putting the first last.*

Conventional Monitoring and Evaluation:

1) *Aims at making a judgment on the program for accountability purposes rather than empowering program stakeholders*

2) *Strives for "scientific" objectivity of M&E findings thereby distancing the external evaluator(s) from stakeholders*

3) *Tends to emphasize the needs for information of program funders and policy makers rather than program implementers and people affected by the program*

4) *Focuses on measurement of success according to predetermined indicators*

(Estrella & Gvanta, 1997; UNFPA, 2004)

Participatory Monitoring and Evaluation:

1. *Is a process of individual and collective learning and capacity development through which people become more aware and conscious of their strengths and weaknesses, their wider social realities, and their visions and perspectives of development outcomes. This learning process creates conditions conducive to change and action.*

2. *Emphasizes varying degrees of participation (from low to high) of different types of stakeholders in initiating, defining the parameters for, and conducting M&E.*

3. *Is a social process of negotiation between people's different needs, expectations, and worldviews. It is a highly political process which addresses issues of equity, power, and social transformation.*

4. *Is a flexible process, continuously evolving and adapting to the program-specific circumstances and needs.*

(Estrella & Gvanta, 1997; UNFPA, 2004)

According to Estrella and Gvanta (1997), there are two principal methods for characterizing participatory monitoring and evaluation (PM&E). The first is by whom the M&E was initiated, and the second is whose perspectives are emphasized. The first determines whether the PM&E is externally or internally led, and the second determines which stakeholders perspectives are emphasized. This is not just speaking of insider versus outsider perspectives; it refers to whose perspectives inside the community are the focus. Many stakeholders may work in partnership to facilitate PM&E, so finding balance between stakeholder perspectives is essential.

Participatory DME for vertical healthcare delivery projects

In vertical healthcare delivery global health initiatives, participatory project design is often about bringing both community stakeholders and local health system stakeholders together in ways that improve those linkages and foster continued follow-up care for recipients of care. Stated another way, we bring vertical and horizontal health programs together to both make improvements in the health of communities and facilitate continuity of care and patient-centered follow-up. In healthcare projects, local healthcare professionals directing volunteers must establish methods for monitoring outcomes.

The End

This ends this book on best practices in global health initiatives. Please share it and make a review if you found the information helpful. If you would like to contact me about speaking or just have questions about the content of this book, you can reach me through our website at info@healthservicecorps.org. In the appendix of this book you will find many resources and links on global health you may find helpful in your cross-cultural work.

Additional Resources

The Institute for Development Studies

http://www.ids.ac.uk/

Results-oriented Monitoring and Evaluation: A Handbook for Programme Managers http://web.undp.org/evaluation/documents/mae-toc.htm

United Nations Population Fund (UNFPA) *Program Manager's Toolkit*

http://www.unfpa.org/monitoring/toolkit.htm

World Vision LEAP Resources - Learning through Evaluation with Accountability and Planning

https://www.wvi.org/sites/default/files/LEAP_2nd_Edition_0.pdf

References

Estrella, M., & Gvanta, J. (1997). *Who counts reality: Participatory monitoring and evaluation.* Brighton, UK: Institute for Development Studies.

UNFPA. (2004). *Program manager's planning and evaluation tool kit:* New York: UN-FPA.

USAID. (1998). *Performance monitoring and evaluation: Guidelines for indicator and data quality.* Washington DC: USAID.

WHO Department of Child and Adolescent Health and Development (CAH). (2004). *Child health in the community.* Geneva: WHO.

WHO Dept. of Child Health and Development. (2009, January). Child and adolescent health topics. Retrieved from http://www.who.int/child_adolescent_health/topics/prevention_care/child/imci/en/

WHO. (2009). *WHO country profiles.* Retrieved from http://www.who.int/countries/en/

WHO Secretary General. (2008). *Progress report on millennium development goals.* New York: United Nations Department of Economic and Social Affairs.

World Vision International, LEAP Team. (2007). *Learning through evaluation with accountability & planning* (2nd ed.). Washington DC: World Vision International.

Chapter 15
Summary and Best Practice in Global Health Resources

I n the early part of this book, we discussed the four general categories of best practices for global health initiatives. Those areas of best practice were patient safety, healthcare system integration and collaboration, facilitation of health development, and community empowerment. We hope the six guidelines set forth in this text provided you some understanding of these respective areas. It should be said at this point that none of us are perfect, and the degree to which respective programs can achieve these best practices varies widely between organizations. It may not be fair to say all six guidelines are expected levels of practice for all volunteer global health programs. However, these six standards remain goals to which all organizations engaged in global health work should aspire. In the beginning of this book, we also talked about five primary ways global health mission work is harmful without adequate knowledge:

6) Without understanding how to maintain patient safety in global health programs, there is great potential for causing actual physical harm to patients.

7) Without wisdom to develop intentional and effective partnership, global health projects often diminish confidence in the local healthcare system and its providers.

8) Without cultural knowledge, global health projects are often paternalistic in nature, offering crisis/temporary relief where long-term development interventions are needed.

9) Without insight into the local context, global health projects often cause economic harm to providers and health systems.

10) Without appropriate perspective, global health projects can be more about making the volunteers happy than the quality of health services provided to care recipients.

We learned that all of these issues can be addressed with study, planning, and willingness to apply standards and guidelines outlined in this text. Addressing patient safety starts with following standards normally adhered to in our home countries and learning those that apply specifically to developing countries. We also learned that there are a number of reasons why patients are at much greater risk of harm from short-term healthcare initiatives than from receiving care in permanent clinics or healthcare facilities. There is no clear or simple answer to patient safety issues, but maintaining focus on safety issues is important for all global initiatives. Strong pre-field global health training is necessary for all international health programs that rely on volunteers. Putting the focus on participatory stakeholder identification, collaboration, and integration can address many of the development concerns around the use of short-term volunteers in global health initiatives.

Participatory program design, monitoring, and evaluation is a fundamental precept of health programming that empowers communities, addresses dependency concerns, and avoids paternalism. The key developmental principle to keep in mind is that short-term global health initiatives are a means, not an end. We must begin to make the shift from activity-oriented initiatives to results-oriented initiatives.

Whether you work with a Christian or strictly humanitarian program, these core principles are the same. They are about finding our way to continuous quality improvement in all four aspects of global health best practices. Some may believe that the concept of volunteers working in global health is itself a contradiction to the idea of best practices. However, we have found that volunteers can be used in a way that truly does represent best practices, but not without focused effort. It is our sincerest prayer that this book can assist you in finding your way to best practices in your global health work.

The rest of this chapter is comprised of additional references you may find helpful.

Additional Standards and Resources for Global health

Child Health

International Standards and Practice Guidelines include the following:

1. WHO child health website

   http://www.who.int/topics/child_health/en/

2. WHO child and adolescent health and development

   http://www.who.int/child_adolescent_health/en/

3. WHO Integrated Management of Childhood Illness (IMCI)

   http://www.who.int/child_adolescent_health/topics/prevention_care/child/imci/en/index.html

4. Model IMCI handbook: Integrated management of childhood illness https://apps.who.int/iris/handle/10665/42939

5. Technical updates of the guidelines on the IMCI http://apps.who.int/iris/bitstream/handle/10665/43303/9241593482.pdf?sequence=1

6. The treatment of diarrhea

   https://www.who.int/publications/i/item/9241593180

7. Management of the child with a serious infection or severe malnutrition

   http://apps.who.int/iris/bitstream/handle/10665/42335/WHO_FCH_CAH_00.1.pdf?sequence=1

8. IMCI Chart Booklet https://cdn.who.int/media/docs/default-source/mca-documents/child/imci-integrated-management-of-childhood-illness/imci-in-service-training/imci-chart-booklet.pdf?sfvrsn=f63af425_1

9. WHO Child Growth Standards https://www.who.int/toolkits/child-growth-standards

10. Inpatient Management of Children with Severe Acute Malnutrition https://apps.who.int/iris/handle/10665/271960

11. Inpatient Management of Acute Malnutrition Training Materials https://www.who.int/publications/i/item/9789240029781

12. Pocket Book of Hospital Care for Children-Guidelines for the Management of Common Illnesses with Limited Resources

    https://www.who.int/publications/i/item/978-92-4-154837-3

13. Emergency Triage Assessment and Treatment (ETAT) course

    https://www.who.int/publications/i/item/9241546875

14. FEAST Trail - Mortality After Fluid Bolus in African Children with Severe Infection

    https://www.nejm.org/doi/full/10.1056/NEJMoa1101549#t=articleResults

Maternal and Newborn Health

International Standards and Practice Guidelines include the following:

1. WHO Maternal Health Website

   http://www.who.int/topics/maternal_health/en/

2. WHO Pregnancy Website

   http://www.who.int/topics/pregnancy/en/

3. WHO Standards for Maternal and Newborn Health

   http://whqlibdoc.who.int/hq/2007/a91272.pdf

4. Making Pregnancy Safer https://www.who.int/europe/activities/making-pregnancy-safer

5. WHO recommended interventions for improving maternal and newborn health
   http://whqlibdoc.who.int/hq/2007/WHO_MPS_07.05_eng.pdf

6.   Pregnancy, childbirth, postpartum and newborn care https://www.who.int/publications/i/item/9789241549356

7.   Managing complications in pregnancy and childbirth

      https://apps.who.int/iris/bitstream/handle/10665/255760/9789241565493-eng.pdf

8.   Managing newborn problems https://apps.who.int/iris/handle/10665/42753

Surgery

International Standards and Practice Guidelines include the following:

1.   WHO Guidelines for Safe Surgery   https://www.who.int/teams/integrated-health-services/patient-safety/research/safe-surgery

2.   Emergency and Essential Surgical Care https://www.who.int/initiatives/who-global-initiative-for-emergency-and-essential-surgical-care

3.   3. Best Practice Guidelines on Emergency Surgical Care in Disaster Situations https://www.who.int/publications/i/item/best-practice-guidelines-on-emergency-surgical-care-in-disaster-situations

4.   4. Surgical Care at the District Hospital - The WHO Manual

      https://apps.who.int/iris/handle/10665/42564

5.   Surgical Safety Check List

      https://www.who.int/teams/integrated-health-services/patient-safety/research/safe-surgery/tool-and-resources

6.   Safe Surgery Saves Lives - The Second Global Safety Challenge

      http://apps.who.int/iris/bitstream/handle/10665/70080/WHO_IER_PSP_2008.07_eng.pdf;jsessionid=48E0230B5E0E6232501C4D4CD-9B70E06?sequence=1

7.   Surgical Site Infection Prevention Guidelines

      https://apps.who.int/iris/bitstream/handle/10665/277399/9789241550475-eng.pdf?sequence=1&isAllowed=y

Resources Listed for Global Health Training

1.   1. Christian Health Service Corps

www.healthservicecorps.org. (Search under resources and courses)

2. 3. Community Toolbox http://ctb.ku.edu/en/default.aspx

3. 4. Global CHE Network http://chenetwork.org/

4. 5. Global Health eLearning Center sponsored by USAID http://www.global-healthlearning.org/

5. 6. Health Education Program for Developing Countries www.hepfdc.info

6. 8. Hesperian Health Guides http://hesperian.org/books-and-resources/

7. 9. Mother and Child Nutrition Protocols http://motherchildnutrition.org/

8. 11. Health Books International https://healthbooksinternational.org/

Disaster Response

International Standards and Practice Guidelines include the following:

1. The Humanitarian Charter and Minimum Standards in Disaster Response of the Sphere Project https://spherestandards.org/handbook-2018/

2. UN OCHA https://www.humanitarianresponse.info/en

3. Humanitarian ID https://auth.humanitarian.id/

4. International Red Cross Red Crescent Code of Conduct https://www.icrc.org/en/doc/resources/documents/publication/p1067.htm

5. WHO health action in crises http://www.who.int/hac/en/

6. WHO health action in crises: Global health cluster https://healthcluster.who.int/

Patient Safety

International Standards and Practice Guidelines include the following:

1. WHO Patient Safety Website

   http://www.who.int/patientsafety/en/

2. Patient Safety Solutions

   https://www.who.int/teams/integrated-health-services/patient-safety/research/patient-safety-solutions

3. WHO Collaborating Centre on Patient Safety Solutions https://www.patientsafetyinstitute.ca/en/About/Programs/WHO-Collaborating-Centre/pages/default.aspx

4. Action on Patient Safety - High 5s

   https://cdn.who.int/media/docs/default-source/patient-safety/high5s/high-5s-action-on-patient-safety.pdf?sfvrsn=1e623c21_6

Development Resources

1. World Vision LEAP Resources - Learning through Evaluation with Accountability and Planning https://www.wvi.org/sites/default/files/LEAP_2nd_Edition_0.pdf

2. The Institute for Development Studies http://www.ids.ac.uk/

3. Results-oriented Monitoring and Evaluation: A Handbook for Programme Managers http://web.undp.org/evaluation/documents/mae-toc.htm

4. United Nations Population Fund (UNFPA) Program Manager's Toolkit

   http://www.unfpa.org/monitoring/toolkit.htm